Testosterone

Editor

KEVIN R. LOUGHLIN

UROLOGIC CLINICS
OF NORTH AMERICA

www.urologic.theclinics.com

Consulting Editor
KEVIN R. LOUGHLIN

November 2022 • Volume 49 • Number 4

ELSEVIER

1600 John F. Kennedy Boulevard • Suite 1800 • Philadelphia, Pennsylvania, 19103-2899

http://www.theclinics.com

UROLOGIC CLINICS OF NORTH AMERICA Volume 49, Number 4
November 2022 ISSN 0094-0143, ISBN-13: 978-0-323-92006-3

Editor: Kerry Holland
Developmental Editor: Diana Ang

Urologic Clinics of North America (ISSN 0094-0143) is published quarterly by Elsevier Inc., 360 Park Avenue South, New York, NY 10010-1710. Months of issue are February, May, August, and November. Business and Editorial Offices: 1600 John F. Kennedy Blvd., Suite 1800, Philadelphia, PA 19103-2899. Periodicals postage paid at New York, NY and additional mailing offices. Subscription prices are $403.00 per year (US individuals), $1054.00 per year (US institutions), $100.00 per year (US students and residents), $459.00 per year (Canadian individuals), $1075.00 per year (Canadian institutions), $100.00 per year (Canadian students/residents), $530.00 per year (foreign individuals), $1075.00 per year (foreign institutions), and $240.00 per year (foreign students/residents). Foreign air speed delivery is included in all *Clinics* subscription prices. All prices are subject to change without notice. **POSTMASTER:** Send address changes to *Urologic Clinics of North America*, Elsevier Health Sciences Division, Subscription Customer Service, 3251 Riverport Lane, Maryland Heights, MO 63043. **Customer Service: 1-800-654-2452 (US). From outside the United States, call 1-314-447-8871. Fax: 1-314-447-8029. E-mail: JournalsCustomerServiceusa@elsevier.com (for print support)** and **JournalsOnlineSupport-usa@elsevier.com (for online support).**

Reprints. For copies of 100 or more, of articles in this publication, please contact the Commercial Reprints Department, Elsevier Inc., 360 Park Avenue South, New York, New York 10010-1710. Tel.: 212-633-3874; Fax: 212-633-3820; E-mail: reprints@elsevier.com.

Urologic Clinics of North America is covered in MEDLINE/PubMed (*Index Medicus*), *Excerpta Medica, Current Contents/Clinical Medicine, Science Citation Index,* and *ISI/BIOMED.*

Contributors

CONSULTING EDITOR

KEVIN R. LOUGHLIN, MD, MBA
Emeritus Professor of Surgery (Urology),
Harvard Medical School, Visiting Scientist,
Vascular Biology Research Program at Boston
Children's Hospital, Boston, Massachusetts,
USA

EDITOR

KEVIN R. LOUGHLIN, MD, MBA
Emeritus Professor of Surgery (Urology),
Harvard Medical School, Visiting Scientist,
Vascular Biology Research Program at Boston
Children's Hospital, Boston, Massachusetts,
USA

AUTHORS

BRADLEY D. ANAWALT, MD
Professor and Vice Chairman, Department of
Medicine, University of Washington, Seattle,
Washington, USA

ANDREW J. ARMSTRONG, MD
Division of Urology, Division of Medical
Oncology, Duke Cancer Institute, Durham,
North Carolina, USA

SHALENDER BHASIN, MB, BS
Professor of Medicine, Harvard Medical
School, Director, Research Program in Men's
Health, Aging and Metabolism, Director,
Boston Claude D. Pepper Older Americans
Independence Center, Boston,
Massachusetts, USA

ARTHUR L. BURNETT, MD, MBA, FACS
Patrick C. Walsh Distinguished Professor of
Urology, Professor, Oncology Center, Johns
Hopkins School of Medicine Brady Urological
Institute, The Johns Hopkins Hospital, Director,
Johns Hopkins Clinical Research Network,
Baltimore, Maryland, USA

LOGAN B. GALANSKY, MD
Johns Hopkins School of Medicine Brady
Urological Institute, The Johns Hopkins
Hospital, Baltimore, Maryland, USA

FRANCESCA F. GALBIATI, MD
Endocrinology Fellow, Division of
Endocrinology, Diabetes, and Hypertension,
Brigham and Women's Hospital, Boston,
Massachusetts, USA

ARIJEET GATTU, MD
Endocrinology Fellow, Division of
Endocrinology, Diabetes, and Hypertension,
Brigham and Women's Hospital, Boston,
Massachusetts, USA

THOMAS GERALD, MD
Fellow, Urologic Oncology, Department of
Urology, The University of Texas Southwestern
Medical Center, Dallas, Texas, USA

ANNA L. GOLDMAN, MD
Assistant Professor of Medicine, Division of
Endocrinology, Diabetes, and Hypertension,

Brigham and Women's Hospital, Boston, Massachusetts, USA

EZGI CALISKAN GUZELCE, MD
Endocrinology Fellow, Division of Endocrinology, Diabetes, and Hypertension, Brigham and Women's Hospital, Boston, Massachusetts, USA

WAYNE J.G. HELLSTROM, MD, FACS
Professor of Urology, Chief of Andrology, Department of Urology, Tulane University School of Medicine, New Orleans, Louisiana, USA

MEHVISH KHAN, MD
Fellow, Division of Endocrinology, Beth Israel Lahey Medical Center, Burlington, Massachusetts, USA

BRENDAN KING, MD
Department of Urology, Tulane University School of Medicine, New Orleans, Louisiana, USA

TOBIAS S. KOHLER, MD, MPH
Department of Urology, Mayo Clinic, Rochester, Minnesota, USA

SRINATH KOTAMARTI, MD
Division of Urology, Duke Cancer Institute, Durham, North Carolina, USA

JASON A. LEVY, DO, MS
Clinical Instructor of Urology, Johns Hopkins School of Medicine Brady Urological Institute, The Johns Hopkins Hospital, Baltimore, Maryland, USA

KEVIN R. LOUGHLIN, MD, MBA
Emeritus Professor of Surgery (Urology), Harvard Medical School, Visiting Scientist, Vascular Biology Research Program at Boston Children's Hospital, Boston, Massachusetts, USA

ANDREW RICHARD MCCULLOUGH, MD
Department of Urology, Co-Director Male Reproductive and Sexual Health, Beth Israel

Lahey Medical Center, Burlington, Massachusetts, USA

ABRAR H. MIAN, BS
Midwestern University, Chicago College of Osteopathic Medicine, Downers Grove, Illinois, USA

ALVARO MORALES, MD, CM, FRCSC, FACS
Department of Urology, Queen's University, Kingston, Ontario, Canada

JUDD W. MOUL, MD
Division of Urology, Duke Cancer Institute, Durham, North Carolina, USA

CALEB NATALE, MD
Department of Urology, Tulane University School of Medicine, New Orleans, Louisiana, USA

THOMAS J. POLASCIK, MD
Division of Urology, Duke Cancer Institute, Durham, North Carolina, USA

GANESH RAJ, MD, PhD
Professor Urology Pharmacology, Paul C. Peters Chair in Urology, Department of Urology, The University of Texas Southwestern Medical Center, Dallas, Texas, USA

D. ROBERT SIEMENS, MD, FRCSC
Department of Urology Queen's University, Kingston, Ontario, Canada

PETER J. SNYDER, MD
Professor of Medicine, Division of Endocrinology, Diabetes and Metabolism, Perelman School of Medicine, University of Pennsylvania, Philadelphia, Pennsylvania, USA

ARTHI THIRUMALAI, MBBS
Section Head of Endocrinology at Harborview Medical Center, Department of Medicine, University of Washington, Seattle, Washington, USA

DAVID Y. YANG, MD
Department of Urology, Emory University, Atlanta, Georgia, USA

Contents

activity, sexual desire, and erectile function; lean body mass, muscle strength, and stair climbing power, and self-reported mobility; areal and volumetric bone mineral density, and estimated bone strength; depressive symptoms; and anemia. Long-term risks of cardiovascular events and prostate cancer during testosterone treatment remain unknown. Testosterone treatment may be offered on an individualized basis to older men with unequivocally low testosterone levels and symptoms or conditions associated with testosterone deficiency after consideration of potential benefits and risks, burden of symptoms, and patient's values.

Testosterone is a steroid hormone that is responsible for the development of normal male sexual characteristics and function as well as the maintenance of homeostasis among multiple organ systems throughout life. Testosterone production is regulated by the hypothalamic-pituitary axis under the direction of gonadotropin-releasing hormone and luteinizing hormone. The testosterone-bound androgen receptor (AR) is a potent regulator of gene expression and may regulate a significant proportion of genes in prostate cells. Therapeutic modulation of testosterone levels and AR signaling activity can be achieved by several different approaches, with distinct consequences and side effects.

Despite newer therapies for castrate-resistant prostate cancer (CRPC), many patients do not experience a treatment response, and most eventually experience secondary resistance. Various androgen-receptor-related and alternative mechanisms of resistance in CRPC have been identified. This focus on understanding the molecular basis of therapeutic resistance, including lineage plasticity, neuroendocrine transformation, and a range of other implicated genomic alterations will hopefully inform decision-making in the care of this lethal cancer.

This article reviews the role of testosterone in normal male sexual anatomic development and function, the consequences of low testosterone on sexual function, and clinical standards for health care providers treating hypogonadal men with sexual dysfunction.

As men age, their serum concentration of total testosterone decreases only slightly, but because the concentration of sex hormone binding globulin increases, the concentration of free testosterone decreases to a greater degree. The testosterone trials demonstrated that testosterone treatment of elderly men who have low serum testosterone levels increases their sexual function, hemoglobin, and bone mineral density to moderate degrees, and their walking, vitality, and mood slightly. Testosterone treatment increases coronary artery noncalcified plaque volume. However, the trials were not large enough or long enough to know if testosterone treatment increases clinical heart disease or prostate disease.

UROLOGIC CLINICS OF NORTH AMERICA

SERIES OF RELATED INTEREST
Surgical Clinics of North America
https://www.surgical.theclinics.com/

Preface

Testosterone: The Hormone of Love, War, and Immortality

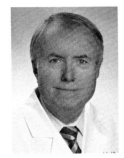

Kevin R. Loughlin, MD, MBA
Editor

Since mankind first appeared on earth, the human psyche has been driven by love, war, and immortality. Through the years, testosterone, both endogenous and exogenous, has been purported to have multiple effects on human behavior and function.

In 1889, Charles-Edouard Brown-Sequard[1] claimed that the injection of a fluid prepared from the testicles of guinea pigs and dogs led to rejuvenation and prolonged human life. It became known as the Brown-Sequard Elixir.

In the early decades of the twentieth century, interest grew in the possibility of testicular transplantation. Lydston[2] and Lespinasse[3,4] reported early attempts with testicular allotransplantation. This was followed by descriptions of xenotransplantation using monkey and goat sources by Voronoff[5] and Brinkley,[6] respectively.

The ongoing understanding of testicular function increased as the Nobel Prize in Chemistry was awarded jointly to Adolf Friedrich Johann Butenandt and Leopold Ruzicka in 1939 for their synthesis of testosterone.[7]

It has been reported that there has been a 58% increase in annual testosterone drug revenue in the United States from 2013 to 2018,[8] and it has been projected that the global hormone replacement therapy market will experience a compound annual growth rate of 7.7% through 2027.[9]

The interest in testosterone therapy has been and continues to be pervasive in both the lay and the medical literature. Testosterone has been considered to have a potential role in sexual function, aggression, and longevity. It has also been investigated for its role in cognition, athletic performance, some malignancies, anemia, and osteoporosis.

With this background, it has been a pleasure to have the opportunity to gather some of the leading experts in the world to review the current state of knowledge on the role of testosterone in clinical medicine for this issue of *Urologic Clinics*. Our understanding of the role of testosterone continues to expand, and this collection of authors provides a current state-of-the-art appraisal of the subject.

Kevin R. Loughlin, MD, MBA
Vascular Biology Program
Boston Children's Hospital
Boston, MA 02115, USA

E-mail address:
kloughlin@partners.org

Urol Clin N Am 49 (2022) ix–x
https://doi.org/10.1016/j.ucl.2022.08.001
0094-0143/22/© 2022 Published by Elsevier Inc.

REFERENCES

1. Brown-Sequard Charles-Edouard. Available at: https://en.wikipedia.org/wiki/Charles-Edouard_Brown-Sequard. Accessed February 12, 2022.
2. Lydston GF. Implantation of generative glands and its therapeutic possibilities. NY Med J 1914;100:745–6.
3. Lespinasse VD. Transplantation of the testicle. J Am Med Assoc 1913;(61):1869–70.
4. Transplantation of the testicle. Chicago Med Recorder 1914;(36):401–3.
5. Voronoff S. Rejuvinating by grafting. London: George Allen and Univ.; 1925. p. 57–60 Imianitoff F, Trans.
6. Brinkley JR. The Brinkley operation. Chicago: Sydney B. Flower; 1922. p. 23.
7. Freeman ER, Bloom DA, McGuire EJ. A brief history of testosterone. J Urol 2001;165(2):371–3.
8. Annual testosterone drug revenue in the U.S. Available at: statistica.com/statistius/320301/predicted-annual-testosterone-drug-revenues-in-the-us/. Accessed February 12, 2022.
9. Hormone replacement therapy market size, share and trends: analysis by product. Available at: https://www.grandviewresearch.com/industry-analysis/hormone-replacement-therapy-market. Accessed February 12, 2022.

The Inexorable March of Prostate Cancer Research
Testosterone and Beyond

Kevin R. Loughlin, MD, MBA

KEYWORDS

- Prostate cancer • Discoveries • Treatments • Surgery • Radiation therapy • Hormonal therapy

KEY POINTS

- The relationship between testosterone and prostate cancer was described by Huggins in 1941.
- Multiple strategies can reduce serum testosterone to castrate levels.
- The observation that some prostate cancers can be observed and that treatment can be deferred was described by Klotz in 2002.
- Genetic testing is playing an increased role in prostate cancer screening and management.
- Immunotherapy and PARP inhibitors are new strategies being pursued for some advanced prostate cancers.

INTRODUCTION

Wikipedia defines a generation as being 20 to 30 years.[1] Although not strictly proven, it has been suggested that surgeons are at their peak from 35 to 55 years of age.[2,3] It therefore should come as no surprise that over the past century or so that, with some noticeable exceptions, major discoveries in prostate cancer treatment have occurred at 20-year intervals.

It can be theorized that each new generation of physicians, surgeons, and nonphysicians alike inherit the knowledge of those who have gone before them. Their own experience accrues, and by the time they reach their professional maturity in their fifties, they have contributed to and added to the knowledge of their field. With this as a construct, the author reviews the history of prostate cancer treatment discoveries over slightly more than the past hundred years.

THE SURGICAL FOUNDATION: HUGH HAMPTON YOUNG, 1904

Although a British surgeon, J. Adams, described the first case of prostate cancer in 1853, Hugh Hampton Young[4] occupies his rightful place as the father of American urology and the father of radical surgery for prostate cancer. In his autobiography, he describes the evolution of his technique of the perineal approach to first remove benign obstruction of the prostate and then radical surgery for prostate cancer.

He performed the first perineal enucleation for benign prostatic obstruction on October 8. 1902. He continued to modify the surgical instruments to enable the perineal approach to prostate surgery, and on April 7, 1904, assisted by William S. Halsted, performed the first radical perineal prostatectomy.[5–8] Through Young's efforts, the perineal approach became the standard approach for radical surgical cure of prostate cancer for much of the remainder of the twentieth century.

THE BRITISH EMPIRE CANCER CAMPAIGN: 1923

Throughout most of the early years of the twentieth century, there was little evidence of collaborative cancer research across institutional lines in either the United States or Europe. A landmark event

Vascular Biology Research Laboratory, Boston Children's Hospital, Harvard Medical School, Boston, MA 02114, USA
E-mail address: kloughlin@partners.org

Urol Clin N Am 49 (2022) 567–572
https://doi.org/10.1016/j.ucl.2022.06.003
0094-0143/22/© 2022 Elsevier Inc. All rights reserved.

urologic.theclinics.com

occurred in 1923 with the establishment of the British Empire Cancer Campaign, which was organized to "attack and defeat the disease of cancer in all its forms, to investigate its causes, distribution, symptoms, pathology and treatment and to promote its cure."

The formation of the British Empire Cancer Campaign provided the underpinning for collaborative science and presaged the formation of the National Cancer Institute by Congress in 1937. As the remainder of the twentieth century unfolded, organized medicine in North America and Europe became increasingly aware of the importance of cancer research.

Also, in the 1930s, Ethel and Alexander Gutman reported that serum acid phosphatase levels increased in patients with metastatic prostate cancer, which became the first and only biomarker for prostate cancer for the next several decades.

CHARLES HUGGINS: THE TESTOSTERONE-PROSTATE CANCER LINK: 1941

It is fair to say that Charles Huggins and the publication of his landmark article on the relationship between prostate cancer and androgens began the modern era of prostate cancer investigation and research.[9] More than 80 years later, androgen deprivation by a variety of means remains the underpinning of the treatment for advanced prostate cancer.[10] As a result of this work, Huggins was awarded the Nobel Prize in Physiology or Medicine in 1966.

THE VETERANS ADMINISTRATION COOPERATIVE UROLOGICAL RESEARCH GROUP STUDIES 1960-1975

Between 1960 and 1975, the Veterans Administration Cooperative Urological Research Group conducted 3 consecutive randomized trials comparing a variety of endocrine treatments for newly diagnosed prostate cancer. These studies, in aggregate, reported 6 major conclusions: (1) An increased hazard of cardiovascular deaths after therapy with 5 mg of diethylstilbestrol (DES); (2) Orchiectomy plus DES was no better than orchiectomy or DES alone; (3) Equivalent effects of 1.0 mg and 5.0 mg DES on prostate cancer; (4) Decreased cardiovascular hazard from therapy with 1.0 mg DES; (5) Premarin and Provera were no better than 1.0 mg DES at the doses studied; (6) Decisions about hormone treatment at diagnosis were dependent on patient characteristics, mainly age and Gleason grade.[11]

DONALD GLEASON: PATHOLOGIC SCORING OF PROSTATE CANCER: 1962

In 1962, Donald Gleason,[12] who was then a young pathologist at the Minneapolis Veterans Administration Hospital, devised the Gleason score, which was an objective, reproducible method to grade prostate cancer. In his obituary, it was mentioned, "The Gleason score has consistently been a key component of our predictive models. It is part of the backbone against which all newer predictive measures have come to be measured."[12]

THE IDENTIFICATION OF PROSTATE-SPECIFIC ANTIGEN: 1970

In the 1960s and 1970s, many researchers were searching for new biomarkers that would facilitate the diagnosis and monitoring of a variety of malignancies.[13] In 1966, Mitsuo Hara[14] reported a partially characterized seminal protein, "gamma-seminoprotein," which was thought to be helpful in rape cases. In 1970, Tien Shun Li and S.J. Behrman,[15] while investigating male infertility, identified antigens in human semen, one of which was later shown to have the same amino acid sequence as prostate-specific antigen (PSA). Also in 1970, Richard Albin identified an antigen that was subsequently identified as PSA.[16] This identification of the association of PSA with prostate tissue, ultimately both benign and malignant, opened up a new era of prostate cancer diagnosis and management.

ANDREW SCHALLY: GONADOTROPIN-RELEASING HORMONE AGONIST ANALOGUES, 1972-1978

Andrew Schally demonstrated that the gonadotropin-releasing hormone (GnRH) agonistic analogue that he and his colleagues had developed between 1972 and 1978 inhibited the growth of prostate cancer in rats. Along with Dr George Tolis, Schally conducted the first clinical trial of GnRH agonists for patients with prostate cancer in 1982. They provided the foundation for this class of drugs to replace orchiectomy or estrogens to achieve castrate levels of serum testosterone. These drugs, as agonists, would initially cause a rise in serum testosterone or a "testosterone flare." Subsequently, GnRH antagonists were developed to obviate the transient testosterone flare. For his work on GnRH agonists, Schally was awarded the Nobel Prize in Physiology or Medicine in 1977.[16]

PATRICK C. WALSH: NERVE-SPARING RADICAL PROSTATECTOMY, 1982

Patrick C. Walsh performed the first nerve-sparing radical nephrectomy in a 52-year-old man at Johns Hopkins Hospital on April 26, 1982. The evolution of his thinking on the practicality of this technique was based on his experience with Pieter Doncker, MD, the outgoing chair of urology in Leiden, The Netherlands. That experience caused Walsh to recognize that the nerves leading to the corpora cavernosa were located outside the capsule and fascia of the prostate. The validation of the technique was confirmed when the patient reported 7 months postoperatively that he had regained potency. The early reports by Walsh ushered in the modern era of nerve-sparing radical prostatectomy as the surgical approach for prostate cancer.[17–19]

MALCOLM BAGSHAW AND RADIATION THERAPY FOR PROSTATE CANCER

Malcolm Bagshaw was the Chief of Radiation Therapy and then Chief of Radiation Oncology at Stanford University from 1960 to 1992. During that time, he introduced radiation therapy, primarily produced by radiation beams generated by a linear accelerator. He established external beam radiation therapy as a viable option for the treatment of localized prostate cancer.

WILLET F. WHITMORE AND INTERSTITIAL IMPLANTATION OF IODINE-125

Willet F. Whitmore is considered by many to be the "father of urologic oncology." Starting in 1970, he began utilizing the open implantation of radioactive iodine-125 seeds with pelvic lymphadenectomy at Memorial Sloan Kettering. Between February 1970 and April 1977, 300 patients with T1, T2, and T3 prostate cancer were treated. The 5-year survival rate for T1-T2 disease was 100% and for T3 was 65%.[20]

LAURENCE KLOTZ AND ACTIVE SURVEILLANCE OF PROSTATE CANCER

Laurence Klotz began enrolling patients with low-risk prostate cancer to an active surveillance protocol starting in 2002.[21] Because of encouraging early results, the enthusiasm for the selective use of active surveillance spread rapidly.

By 2018, Klotz reported that there had been 2400 publications on the topic of active surveillance in prostate cancer with more than 20,000 patients reported in the prospective series.[22] The use of active surveillance for management of prostate

cancer has been increasing significantly. Using data from the Surveillance, Epidemiology, and End Results Program–Medicare, Liu and colleagues[23] reported that the use of active surveillance increased from 22% in 2004 to 2005 to 50% in 2014 to 2015 in patients with a Gleason score of 6 or below and increased from 9% in 2004 to 2005 to 13% in 2014 to 2015 for patients with a Gleason score of 7 or above.[23] The intensity of the surveillance, including biomarkers, imaging and biopsies, continues to evolve.[24]

LAPAROSCOPIC AND ROBOTIC PROSTATECTOMY

Laparoscopic prostatectomy was introduced in 1991 and began to become more widely utilized over the next decade.[25] However, it was not until 2008 when robotic prostatectomy began being introduced into urologic practice.[26] Tyson and colleagues[27] reviewed radical prostatectomy trends in the United States over a 14-year period. They found an overall decrease of 7% in the total number of prostatectomies during that period. That trend was likely due, at least in part, to an increased enthusiasm for active surveillance and a greater acceptance of radiation therapy with a lead in of androgen ablation.[24] It was significant that the number of open prostatectomies decreased by 70% during that time, and 18% of hospitals stopped performing open prostatectomies altogether.[26,27]

They further reported that from 2008 to 2011, the number of laparoscopic radical prostatectomies declined by 90%, and the number of open radical prostatectomies declined by 50%.[26,27] Similar trends were reported by Lowrance and colleagues[28] utilizing case logs from the American Board of Urology.

THE ANTIANDROGENS

As mentioned previously, the work of Huggins provided the initial foundation for the relationship between testosterone and prostate cancer. As research continued throughout the twentieth century, the key role of the androgen receptor came to be recognized and better understood.

A class of drugs known collectively as first-generation androgen receptor inhibitors, including flutamide, bicalutamide, and nilutamide, was introduced clinically in the last 2 decades of the twentieth century.[29] These drugs target androgen receptor translocation to the nucleus and prevent downstream signaling. Cyproterone acetate is another antiandrogen but has not been available in the United States. The second-generation antiandrogens began with enzalutamide in 2012 and was followed by apalutamide and darolutamide, to improve on the mechanism. Abiraterone acetate prevents androgen biosynthesis.[30]

These drugs have been studied in a series of double-blind, placebo-controlled trials for efficacy and safety of these drugs in nonmetastatic castration-resistant prostate cancer. These trials revealed that enzalutamide (PROSPER Trial) and apalutamide (SPARTAN Trial) and darolutamide (ARAMIS Trial) improved survival in high-risk, nonmetastatic castration-resistant prostate cancer, and darolutamide may result in fewer adverse results.[31] This class of drugs is now part of the clinical armamentarium for treating selected patients with high-risk prostate cancer.

PROSTATE BIOPSY TECHNIQUES

The technique of prostate imaging and biopsy techniques has evolved and continues to undergo evolution. Over the past century, biopsy by digital palpation, ultrasound guidance, and MRI guidance have all been utilized by the urologic community. Controversy continues over the number of cores, antibiotic prophylaxis, and optimal imaging techniques. A detailed discussion of these issues is beyond the scope of this article, and the reader is referred to the current American Urological Association White Paper on the topic.[32]

GENETIC TESTING AND PROSTATE CANCER RISK

Over recent years, there have been increasing applications of genetic testing to evaluate prostate cancer risk. The Philadelphia Prostate Cancer Consensus Conference was convened to investigate this topic. At the conclusion of this conference, the following recommendations were made: Large, germline panels and somatic testing were recommended for metastatic prostate cancer. Reflex testing–initial testing of priority genes followed by expanded testing was suggested for multiple scenarios. Metastatic disease or family history suggestive of hereditary prostate cancer was recommended for germline testing. Priority genes to test for metastatic disease treatment included BRCA 2, BRCA 1, and mismatch repair genes with broader testing, such as ATM, for clinical trial eligibility. BRCA 2 was recommended for active surveillance discussions. Screening starting at age 40 years or 10 years before the youngest prostate cancer diagnosis in a family was recommended for BRCA 2 carriers, with consideration in HOXB13, BRCA2, ATM, and mismatch repair carriers.[33]

BIOMARKERS

Over the past several decades, there has been a panoply of prostate cancer biomarkers. These include serum, urine, and tissue biomarkers, which have been utilized for diagnosis, surveillance, and prognosis. This is beyond the scope of this article, but excellent recent reviews are available.[34,35]

IMMUNOTHERAPY AND PROSTATE CANCER

In 2018, James P. Allison and Tasuku Honjo were awarded the Nobel Prize in Physiology or Medicine for their discovery of cancer therapy by inhibition of negative immune regulation. The role of immunotherapy in the treatment of prostate cancer is still in its nascent, but exciting stage. Multiple treatment strategies are being pursued, including tumor infiltrating lymphocytes, vaccine-based therapies, CTLA-4 inhibition, PD-1, PDL-1 inhibition, CTLA-4/PD-1 combination, bispecific T-cell engagers, and chimeric antigen receptor T-cell therapy.[36] There are now several phase III clinical trials underway that are evaluating the use of checkpoint inhibitors in a variety of prostate cancer circumstances. The next few years hold the promise of introducing an era of exciting new discoveries.

POLY(ADENOSINE DIPHOSPHATE-RIBOSE) POLYMERASE INHIBITORS AND PROSTATE CANCER

Germinal and/or somatic alterations of the DNA-damage response pathway genes were found in a substantial number of patients with advanced prostate cancers, mainly of poor prognosis. These alterations induce a dependency for single-strand break reparation through the poly(adenosine diphosphate-ribose) polymerase (PARP) system, which provided the rationale to develop PARP inhibitors.[37]

PARP is a family of 17 distinct proteins in which PARP 1 and 2 are involved in DNA repair. PARP 1 binds to damaged DNA gaps, and after conformational change, induces PARylation. PARP inhibitors are oral targeted therapies that competitively bind to NAD+ sites of PARP 1 and PARP 2, inducing a catalytic inhibition. Five different molecules are currently under development or recently approved: olaparib, rucaparib, niraparib, veliparib, and talazoparib. Their action inhibits the PARylation, and therefore, single-strand DNA break repair. These ongoing studies will provide important information about the role of PARP inhibitors in clinical medicine.

PROSTATE CANCER RESEARCH: THE MODERN ERA

It is fair to say that there have been several eras in prostate cancer research. The ground-breaking research of Huggins in the 1940s provided the underpinning for the understanding of the role of testosterone in the development of prostate cancer. The period from 1982 to 2002 may well be considered to be the Localized Prostate Cancer Era. The period from 2002 until now may be considered the Indolent Prostate Cancer Era. Now it would appear that we are entering the Prostate Cancer Genetics and Metastatic Prostate Cancer Era.

The next 20 years hold great promise for prostate cancer treatment. The collaborative research of urologists, radiation oncologists, medical oncologists, endocrinologists, and basic scientists will undoubtedly result in major clinical breakthroughs that will benefit our patients.

CLINICS CARE POINTS

- The role of serum and intraprostatic androgen levels continues to be a topic of intense investigation.
- Continued biomarker development, including genetic testing in selected patients, will aid both diagnosis and management of patients with prostate cancer.
- Selection of treatments for localized prostate cancer needs to be individualized according to the patient's characteristics, the tumor's characteristics, and the wishes of the patient and his family.

REFERENCES

1. Generation. Available at: En.wikipedia.org/wiki/generation. Accessed March 14, 2022.
2. Surgeons reach peak performance between 35 and 50. Daily Mail Reporter 2012.
3. Duclus A, Peix J-L, Colin C. Influence of experience on performance of individual surgeons in thyroid surgery: prospective cross sectional multicentre study. BMJ 2012;344.
4. Young HH. Hugh Young: a surgeon's autobiography. New York: Harcourt, Brace and Company; 1940. p. 106.
5. About Dr. Hugh H. Young, chairman 1897-1941, Brady Urological Institute, Johns Hopkins Medicine. Available at: hopkinsmedicine.org/brady-urology-institute-about_us/history_of_urology_at_johns_hopkins. Accessed March 15, 2022.
6. British Empire Cancer Campaign. Available at: Welcome.collection.org/works/u917m4cs. Accessed March 15, 2022.
7. Gutman EB, Sproul EE, Gutman AB. Significance of increased phosphatase activity of bone at the site of osteoblastic metastases secondary to carcinoma of the prostate gland. Am J Cancer 1936; 28:485–95.
8. Gutman AB, Gutman EB. An 'acid' phosphatase occurring in the serum of patients with metastasizing carcinoma of the prostate gland. J Clin Invest 1938; 17:473–8.
9. Huggins C, Hodges CV. Studies on prostate cancer 1. The effect of castration, of estrogen, and of androgen injection on serum phosphatases in metastatic carcinoma o the prostate. Cancer Res 1941; 1(4):293–7.
10. Albertsen P. Androgen deprivation in prostate cancer-step by step. N Engl J Med 2009;360: 2572–4.
11. Byar DP, Carle DK. Hormone therapy for prostate cancer: results of the Veterans Administration cooperative research group studies. NCI Monogr 1788;7: 165–70.
12. Obituary-Donald F. Gleason. Lancet 2009;373:540.
13. Catalona W. History of the discovery and clinical translation of prostate specific antigen. Asian J Urol 2014;1(1):12–4.
14. Hara M, Inove T, Koyanagi Y. Preparation and immunoelectrophoretic assessment of antisera to human seminal plasma. Nippon Haigajku Zasshi 1966;20: 356–60.
15. Li TS, Behrman SJ. The sperm and seminal plasma-specific antigens of human semen. Fert Steril 1970; 21:565–73.
16. Albin RJ, Soanes WA, Bronson P, et al. Precipitating antigens of the normal human prostate. Reprod Fertil 1970;22:573–4.
17. The William P. Didusch Center For Urologic Surgery, The American Urological Association. Available at: urologichistorymuseum/histories/people-in-urology/w/Patrick-craig-walsh#. Accessed March 15, 2022.
18. White T. Malcolm Bagshaw, pioneer in developing radiation therapies for cancer, dies at 86. Stanford Med News 2011.
19. Loughlin KR. The Whitmore aphorism. Urol Oncol 2018;36(11):473–4.
20. Sogani PC, Whitmore WF, Hilaris BS, et al. Experience with inherited implantation of iodine-125 in the treatment of prostatic carcinoma. Scand J Urol Nephrol 1980;55:205–11.
21. Klotz L. Active surveillance with selective delayed intervention: a biologically nuanced approach to favorable-risk prostate cancer. Clin Prost Cancer 2003;2(2):106–10.

22. Klotz L. The future of active surveillance. Transl Androl Urol 2018;7(2):256–9.

23. Liu Y, Hall IJ, Filson C, et al. Trends in the use of active surveillance and treatments in Medicare beneficiaries diagnosed with localized prostate cancer. Urol Oncol 2021;39(7):432–7.

24. Loughlin KR. The hammer and nail phenomenon: the expanding acceptance of active surveillance in urologic oncology. Urol Oncol 2021;39(5):281–5.

25. Schuessler WW, Schulam PG, Clayman RV, et al. Laparoscopic radical prostatectomy: initial short-term experience. Urology 1997;58(6):854–7.

26. Dalela D, Menon M. Re: Contemporary trends in radical prostatectomy in the United States: open versus minimally invasive surgery 1998-2011. Mayo Clin Proc 2016;91(1):1–2.

27. Tyson MD, Andrews PE, Ferrigni RF, et al. Contemporary trends in radical prostatectomy in the United States 1998-2011. Mayo Clin Proc 2016;91(1):10–6.

28. Lowrance WT, Eastman JA, Savage C, et al. Contemporary and robotic radical prostatectomy practice patterns among urologists in the United States. J Urol 2012;187(6):2087–92.

29. Estebanez-Perpina E, Bevan CL, McEwan IJ. Eighty years of targeting androgen receptor activity in prostate cancer: the fight goes on. Cancers(Basel) 2021; 13(3):509–28.

30. Rice MA, Malhotra SV, Stoyanova T. Second generation antiandrogens: from discovery to standard of care in castrate resistant prostate cancer. Front Oncol 2019;9:801–28.

31. Hird AE, Magee DE, Bhindi B, et al. A systematic review and network meta-analysis of novel androgen receptor inhibitors in non-metastatic castration-resistant prostate cancer. Clin Genitourinary Cancer 2020;18(5):343–50.

32. Taneja SS, Bjurlin MA, Carter HB et al. American Urological Association, Inc. AUA/Optimal Techniques of Prostate Biopsy Specimen Handling 2014. Available at: auanet.org/guidelines/prostate-needle-bioposy-complications. Accessed March 15, 2022.

33. Giri VN, Knudsen KE, Kelly WK, et al. Implementation of genetic testing for prostate cancer: Philadelphia prostate cancer consensus conference 2019. J Clin Oncol 2020;38(24):2798–811.

34. Porzycki P, Ciskowicz E. Modern biomarkers in prostate cancer diagnosis. Cent Eur J Urol 2020;73(3): 300–6.

35. Duffy MJ. Biomarkers for prostate cancer: prostate-specific antigen and beyond. J Clin Chem Lab Med 2020;58(3):326–39.

36. Fay EK, Graff JN. Immunotherapy in prostate cancer. Cancers(Basel) 2020;12(7):1752. https://doi.org/10.3390/cancers1207/1752.

37. Teyssonneau D, Margot H, Cabart M, et al. Prostate cancer and PARP inhibitors: progress and challenges. J Hemat Oncol 2021;14(51). https://doi.org/10.1186/s13045-021-01061.

Testosterone Therapy and Prostate Cancer
Incorporating Low-Level Evidence into Practical Recommendations

Alvaro Morales, MD, CM, FRCSC*, D. Robert Siemens, MD, FRCSC[1]

KEYWORDS

- Testosterone therapy • Exogenous androgens • Prostate cancer

KEY POINTS

- For almost 80 years, the use of exogenous androgens was considered an absolute contraindication in men with prostate cancer. Over the last 2 decades additional experience has shown that this view was too rigid and that under specific circumstances some flexibility is warranted.
- Consideration for testosterone therapy for men with prostate cancer should be limited to those with a clinical picture and laboratory confirmation of hypogonadism
- Hypogonadal men successfully treated for prostate cancer are candidates for testosterone therapy. Those on active surveillance and low risk disease are also candidates as long as long as some requirements are met. Recurrent prostate cancer or high risk of recurrence may be candidates under very specific conditions.
- All these patients require close and competent follow with initial and periodic evaluation including pertinent laboratory determinations.

INTRODUCTION

In men's health 2 fields share the characteristics of being both controversial and involving several medical disciplines: testosterone deficiency syndrome (TDS) and prostate cancer (PCa). Although Geriatrics, Endocrinology, Oncology, and Family Medicine could rightly assume some responsibilities in the care of men with TDS and PCa, urologists manage the vast majority of men diagnosis of PCa. Equally, Urology plays a preponderant role in dealing with male hypogonadism.

THE CONTROVERSY

Early in this century, a polemic emerged on the interactions between androgens and PCa development and progression. Former beliefs dating back 8 decades were vigorously questioned and newly refined and increasingly accepted. However, the deeply ingrained concerns about the safety of testosterone (T) administration to men with, or at risk, of PCa remain conspicuous.

ANDROGENS AND PROSTATE CANCER

Shortly after the synthesis of testosterone (T)[1,2] studies established a vital role in the development and function of the prostate. Since then, much progress has been made on the relationships between T and prostate health. Research resulted in the revision of early concepts and firmly held views were challenged following discoveries in the disciplines of biochemistry, genetics, and immunology. Developments in the understanding of the interactions between androgens and the androgen receptor (AR)[3–6] and the concept of the prostate being an endocrine organ within the hypothalamus–pituitary–gonadal axis[7,8] as well as the determination of intracrine steroidogenesis in

Department of Urology Queen's University, Kingston, Ontario, Canada
[1] Present address: 76 Stuart St. Kingston, Ontario K7L 2V7, Canada.
* Corresponding author. 1205–1000 King Street West, Kingston, Ontario K7M 8H3, Canada.
E-mail address: moralesa@queensu.ca

Urol Clin N Am 49 (2022) 573–582
https://doi.org/10.1016/j.ucl.2022.07.002
0094-0143/22/© 2022 Elsevier Inc. All rights reserved.

benign and malignant prostate tissues,[9] translated into a wealth of information on the interrelations and clinical significance of hormones in prostate health. The finding of intricate intraindividual and intratumoral genomic and phenotypic heterogeneity of PCa provided a better understanding of the complexity of this neoplasm and its treatment.[10]

Evolving progress, such as the elucidation of the role of extracellular vesicles capable of transferring functional molecules over significant distances,[11,12] as well as the documentation that androgen deprivation therapy (ADT) alters the gut microbiota resulting in a buildup of bacterial species capable of synthetizing androgens thus promoting the progression of castration resistance PCa (CRPC)[13] have diagnostic and therapeutic repercussions. The identification of dormancy, that PCa uniquely shares with estrogen receptor-positive breast cancer, is in infancy but offers the clarification of poorly defined mechanisms in the evolution of PCa.[14]

THE ANDROGEN RECEPTOR AND THE PROSTATE

An essential player in the translation of androgen action is the AR, a nuclear transcription factor with distinctive molecular features that binds to androgens and acts through differential DNA targeting and genetic control on the relevant organ systems.[15] On binding to the AR in the prostate, T acts mostly as a prohormone. The effective androgen is the more potent dihydrotestosterone (DHT). The variance in the potency of T versus DHT is due to DHT much slower dissociation times, a concept with profound therapeutic implications.[16] The effects of androgens on the prostate are unquestionable although not yet fully characterized.[17] The glandular epithelium is the primary androgen target within the gland. DHT acts on the ARs of these tissues to generate a variety of peptide growth factors leading to mitogenic effects and divergence of survival signaling (apoptosis).[18] Androgen deprivation, results in insufficient production of andromedins that signals the apoptotic cascade in the secretory compartment of the prostatic epithelium.[19] Understanding the mechanisms of androgen-dependent prostate cells growth, differentiation and death are important because their manipulation has major consequences in the management of PCa[20] (discussed in detail in section 5 of this issue).

ANDROGENS HOMEOSTASIS AND PROSTATE CANCER RISK

Despite the absence of contemporary evidence, there remains a deep-rooted perception that androgens play a substantial causal role in the development of PCa. This is not surprising considering these known tenets about T and the prostate gland:

- At puberty in the presence of profound hypogonadism, the prostate fails to develop.[21]
- The intuitive hypothesis that low endogenous T levels prevent or delay the incidence and progression of PCa as shown by the results of cancer prevention trials, including finasteride in PCPT.[22]
- Reports on serum T levels associated with PCa diagnosis, including the high prevalence of biopsy detectable prostate cancer (PCa) in men with low testosterone.[23,24]
- The increase in PSA values following androgen stimulation[25]
- The favorable impact of adjuvant ADT with radiotherapy and some early evidence of benefit of neoadjuvant intense ADT in men with high-risk PCa.[26]
- The outstanding, though often temporary, the response of patients to ADT and to the more recently introduced AR targeted therapies in men with advanced disease.[27]

It is, therefore, not surprising that there is a belief among clinicians that low serum T prevents or, delays the development of PCa. By extension, once it has developed, it would progress at a slower rate in a hypogonadal milieu. Reports on the discovery of "occult" PCa shortly after the initiation of TTh further reinforce the concept of a positive correlation between androgens and PCa development and growth.[28,29]

As any other solid tumor, PCa is the result of a chain of genetic and epigenetic mutations resulting in abnormal cell signaling pathways promoting their immortality. For each cancer these mutations define the interactions of the tumor with its immediate microenvironment.[30] For PCa, its relations with the hormonal microenvironment are of crucial importance. Credit must be given to the pioneering work of Huggins, including his prescient observation about bipolar therapy: "In hormone-dependent cancers, the supporting hormones are of cardinal importance in maintaining the life of the malignant cell. This is the principle of cancer control by hormone deprivation. Cancers can also be controlled by supplying large amounts of hormones; this is the principle of hormone interference."[31] Decades later, Labrie[32] demonstrated that PCa cells are capable of producing potent androgens (T and DHT) from less powerful precursors such as dehydroepiandrosterone (DHEA). It is now clearly established that in addition to the endocrine processes involving gonadal steroids the intracrine pathways are significant participants in PCa promotion.[33–35]

RELEVANT CLINICAL SITUATIONS

A contributing factor to some of the controversial issues involving the interactions between androgens and PCa stem from the ambiguity of the clinical situations under discussion. There are 3 pertinent clinical situations:

Hypogonadal Men Without the Evidence of Prostate Cancer

It has been determined and broadly accepted that men with a clinical picture of hypogonadism *and* biochemical confirmation of abnormally low T are candidates for TTh.[36] Unfortunately, a significant number of men are reportedly prescribed T without having basic laboratory evaluations[37] and sometimes for flimsy clinical evidence as a cure-all for the infirmities of aging. Guidelines by recognized specialty societies, universally concur[36–38] with the need for baseline investigations. There is no justification for giving T without ruling out potentially serious health issues that may further deteriorate as a consequence T treatment.[39]

Contemporary recommendations, regarding prostate health, are that symptomatic hypogonadal men can safely receive TTh.[36–38,40] Monitoring during treatment includes the requirement of baseline documentation by a digital rectal examination (DRE) as well as a measurement of prostatic specific antigen (PSA). It is also recommended that these should be repeated every 3 months during the first year of TTh and yearly thereafter.

Hypogonadal Men Successfully Treated for Cancer of the Prostate (CaP)

Technically these men would be classified in the previous category, the reality is different and still evolving. There is a significant body of evidence indicating that they are candidates for TTh:

- Still inconclusive but compelling evidence showing that following radical prostatectomy, men with symptomatic hypogonadism can safely receive supplemental T.[41,42]
- Smaller but equally encouraging evidence has been presented for similar patients treated with either brachytherapy[43] or external beam radiotherapy.[44,45]
- Studies supporting these views warn that the findings are hypothesis-generating and require confirmation with multicenter controlled trials.[46]

A paramount concern in this scenario focuses on the timing TTh; it has not been established but has been vaguely described as "after a prudent interval".[47] This, of course, is of limited help to the clinician. It is our belief (without much evidence to support it) that for those who underwent radical prostatectomy the "prudent interval" is achieved once the PSA is no longer detectable. Consideration must be given to the histopathological information of the surgical specimen (grade group, margins, stage). We advocated for a potential advantage of the early initiation of T supplementation in that an elevation of the PSA may indicate incomplete ablation of cancer, in which case additional curative measures may be considered; something akin to a challenge test[48]. This concept received support at the 2021 AUA meeting whereby Mulhall and colleagues[49] reported on a prospective study of hypogonadal men who had undetectable PSA after radical prostatectomy and were challenged with T administration. Persuasively, those who had an elevation of the PSA following TTh (10%), had detectable disease on imaging.

The situation is more complex for those with low or intermediate PCa who underwent radiotherapy without ADT as undetectable PSA levels might not be attainable. For these men, we would consider the initiation of T treatment after a persistent PSA nadir (>6 months) has been reached.

This cohort demands a close and competent follow-up, particularly in the initial months of TTh. There is no justification to initiate TTh without baseline determinations including T and PSA which are reported not being measured in about 30% of patients in this category in the United States.[50] Monitoring is equally important and frequently ignored.[51]

Hypogonadal Men with Active CaP

Opinions about treating hypogonadism in men undergoing active management of PCa are the most controversial and, the least backed with reliable experimental or clinical information. Despite some anecdotal fulsome views,[52] the use of TTh in men with PCa requires the consideration of the complexity of the tumor's biological behavior in relation to androgens. Those interactions were described above, but they become vastly more intricate when considering the emergence of androgen independence by PCa.

Processes of resistance to ADT can either be mediated by the AR or by other mechanisms that bypass it (comprehensively reviewed by Crawley and colleagues).[53] In addition, preclinical models suggest that AR overexpression represents a therapeutic liability that can be exploited with reinstitution of the ligand to promote cell death[54,55] and constitute examples of the intricate connections between androgens and the AR in PCa.

In our estimation, there are 3 distinct cohorts of men with PCa and symptomatic hypogonadism who are potential candidates for TTh but need to be considered separately.

a) Those who have been diagnosed as harboring a localized PCa but whom, for a variety of reasons remain untreated

Treatment options for these men have been detailed in the AUA.ASTRO/SUO guideline.[56] The document, does not contemplate the situation of men who, concomitantly with PCa, endure troublesome hypogonadism. In the absence of more reliable information it is suggested that.

- For those with low-risk diseases, active surveillance (AS) is currently the preferred recommendation. We would add that if a man is on AS and is hypogonadal justifying treatment, he is a potential candidate for TTh if the conditions listed (**Boxes 1** and **2**) are met.
- For those with intermediate- and high-risk disease that chose watchful waiting rather than active management due to personal choice and/or comorbidity, the manifestations of hypogonadism would have to be sufficiently severe and disabling to merit TTh. However, if these unique and relatively uncommon circumstances are present, it is our view that criteria shown in the tables and algorithm should apply.[57] These men should be encouraged to participate in a clinical registry.

b) Recurrent PCa or at high risk of recurrence after treatment with curative intent

This is a challenging cohort as the development of TD in these men may be associated with the initial treatment (radiotherapy, lack of T recovery after adjuvant ADT) or may have pre-existed the finding of PCa. In the majority, hypogonadism is of limited importance as the symptoms may not be necessarily related to their androgen levels but more closely linked to aspects raised by the diagnosis and treatment of the PCa and the worrisome prognosis when facing an initial treatment failure[58,59]

The need for TTh in these men requires exceptional considerations. The indications for it would depend on multiple factors including details of their original tumor and time as its management as well as the plan for the additional treatment of unresolved cancer, one of which would be to establish an even more profound hypogonadal environment aiming at castrate levels of T.[60] It is our perspective that to be considered a candidate for TTh in this situation, the manifestations of hypogonadism should be florid, incapacitating and supported by laboratory confirmation of low serum T,[61] an opinion not universally accepted.[62] Short-acting preparations should be used, particularly in the early phase of T administration, as a prudent approach in case of an exacerbation of the PCa.[63]

c) Those in whom PCa developed resistance to castrate levels of T

Unfortunately, the development of CRPC is a common event in advanced PCa, secondary to multiple mechanisms including the upregulation of the AR from sustained hypogonadism.[9]

For these men, rapid cycling between high and low levels of serum T known as bipolar androgen therapy (BAT) has been investigated with promising results.[64,65] This model is the result of solid empirical observations[66,67] and illustrates the appropriate methodical approach to changing paradigms: well-designed clinical trials such as TRANSFORMER,[68] which are already providing early hopeful answers and others like BAT-RAD starting enrollment in early 2022.[69] Managing patients with the BAT template should be carried out by experienced multi-disciplinary teams under an investigational protocol. Referral to clinical trials for men failing standard chemotherapy or novel androgen target therapies should be encouraged.

DISSECTING THE CONTROVERSY: PAST, PRESENT, AND FUTURE

Viewpoints endorsing the administration of exogenous T to hypogonadal men with PCa cite low-level evidence suggesting that little, if any tumor progression occurs following T administration: "in selected cases" providing TTh to men with metastatic disease is not equivalent to "pouring gasoline on a fire".[70] We first reported[71] on observations in a group of men with CRPC primed with T before receiving intravenous radioactive phosphorus for control of severe bone pain from metastatic disease. Most of these men experienced an exacerbation of related signs and symptoms although a small number (14%) had a temporary remission on T alone. We did not have an explanation for this observation until Fowler and Whitmore[72] suggested the notion of the "saturation model" (SM). Briefly, it proposes that changes in T concentrations below the point of maximal AR binding will enhance PCa growth. In contrast, once maximal AR binding is reached

Box 1
Criteria to consider before initiating TTh in a patient with TD and PCa

- An experienced, qualified, and interested physician
- A patient able and willing to provide informed consent
- An engaged patient committed to a shared-decision making process
- A clinical picture supporting the diagnosis of significant hypogonadism
- Serum T levels supporting the diagnosis of TD
- Absence of spinal metastases with risk of cord compression
- Absence of contraindications for TTh (eg, erythrocytosis, congestive heart failure)
- Favor short-acting T formulations in the early period of treatment
- A priori settlement of benchmarks for the cessation of TTh (eg, PSA velocity/increase ≥ 20% within first 3 months)
- Contemplate referral/participation in a clinical trial, registry

the presence of additional androgens results in negligible additional effect.

Their observations shared our finding that the large majority of patients (>80%) receiving T experienced unfavorable responses but also that a prompt regression of these undesirable effects occurs on the withdrawal of T.[73] The intriguing findings remained unexplored for decades but have been revived, expanded and promoted.[74–76]

Morgentaler and colleagues[77] published a collective experience of 2 institutions whereby 13

Box 2
Basic evaluations at onset and during TTh in a hypogonadal man with PCa

- Evaluation of functional response to TTh at 3 and 6 months
- Baseline hematology and biochemistry (serum T, hematocrit, hemoglobin, PSA)
- Imaging for the documentation of loco-regional or metastatic disease depending on the specific oncological scenario
- Follow-up hematology and biochemistry monthly for initial 3 months and every 3 to 6 months thereafter, if stable

men who received TTh while on active surveillance for lower risk PCa: not only there was no evidence of progression of their disease and follow-up biopsies were negative for cancer in over half of the patients. Simultaneously, we[66] reported observations in a comparable group of 7 men but our outcomes were different. Although some of them did well, there was marked inconsistency in the response to TTh and the response was unpredictable. The finding of significant inter-individual responses to changes in the hormonal milieu of men with PCa is not surprising considering that multiple genomic, transcriptomic phenotypic, and epigenetic heterogeneity are present not only among individuals but also within the same individual.[10,78] There is also the age differential in the aromatization of T,[79] the diverting kinetics of the 2 isoforms of 5 α-reductase[16] and the changes occurring in the AR signaling pathways during prostate carcinogenesis[80] translating in inconsistencies in the response of PCa to T.

The reintroduction and widespread attention given to the saturation model has the potential to lead to the relaxation of former paradigms regarding the use TTh in men with PCa. However, eschewing more cautious guidelines from professional medical associations[36–38] may be premature for a variety of reasons:

1. The saturation model is not a universally accepted construct. In fact, serious questions have been raised about its validity.[81]
2. Significant limitations of studies supporting it include their retrospective and single-arm design, inadequate power, insufficient follow-up, and the heterogeneity of the baseline characteristics of the participants[82]
3. Despite the number of small positive observational studies there is a paucity of information on crucial clinical endpoints such as metastasis-free survival, or other important progression events in men with PCa receiving TTh.[83]
4. The now well-recognized heterogeneity of PCa may translate into similar heterogeneity in aggressiveness and potential progression as a result of TTh[77,84,85]
5. All previous reports attempting to mitigate concerns about the use of T in men with CaP include specific warnings that the results are preliminary, hypothesis generating, and requiring more investigation to demonstrate efficacy and unequivocal safety[46,86]
6. An extensive systematic search from 1941 to 2019, revealed that TTh is detrimental to patients with advanced PCa (progression rate of at least 38.5%) as well as for those with treated

high-risk disease successfully treated for (14.4%–57.1%)[87]

7. There is an ongoing, alarming lack of pertinent detail focused on critical clinical issues to help direct safe utilization of TTh in patients with PCa: (a) baseline patient and cancer characteristics; (b) timing for the onset/discontinuation of TTh; (c) formulations of T to use; (d) standards of follow-up (frequency of assessments and nature of the evaluations (ie, biochemistry, hematology).[78] Little has changed in this regard in the last 2 decades[88]

To tackle time-honored "myths" on the use of T in men *known to have* PCa convincingly, we need ethically approved, properly sponsored, well-designed, rigidly controlled, and carefully monitored studies. Otherwise, the use of T in these men may be construed as reckless in a field already beleaguered by controversy.

The prevalence of hypogonadal men aged 40 to 69 years old who are potential candidates for T administration is projected to reach 481,000 new cases by 2025 in the USA,[89] This, is a vastly larger population than any cohort of men diagnosed with PCa. Thus, there is a very limited number of cases for the conduction of validation studies by single institutions. Registries such as CapSURE[90] are the obvious answer and work appropriately at national levels. There is, however, a large global population of potential candidates that could amplify and solidify the national experiences and that could be reached with a straightforward and universally accessible protocol.[72]

SUMMARY

Current evidence strongly supports that hypogonadal men successfully treated for PCa can safely receive TTh. For those harboring untreated PCa the picture is less clear as this group of men undoubtedly expands due to acceptance of AS as the preferred initial treatment strategy[91] and experience increases with emerging technologies such as MRI and genomic testing,[92–94] prostate-specific membrane antigen PSMA theranostics,[95] and fear of complications or regret of treatment choices.[96]

There is a lack of guiding criteria for the general urologist who should be cautious and embark on it with a great deal of thoughtfulness. For untreated PCa there must be strong valid reasons for not moving forward to curative treatment and an equally strong one for TTh. For the unsuccessfully treated, BAT is a promising oncological option although requires much more prospective study given the ever-changing landscape of CRPC.

Urology should strive for higher levels of evidence, such as clinical registries or other correlative observations from prospective trials, to characterize those clinical scenarios whereby men with TDS and PCa would benefit most from TTh in terms of quality of life. The considerations that we must take into account include the specific baseline patient and cancer characteristics as well as the particular stage in their cancer journey. In addition, we should endeavor to establish the criteria to initiate/discontinue TTh, requirements for follow-up, and T formulations to use. These are essential needs for wide acceptance of the evolving paradigm.

ILLUSTRATIVE CASES

1. A 60-year-old healthy man is referred for a second opinion regarding known TD before his radical prostatectomy for PCa 1 year ago. He was interested in discussing going back on TTh. Initial PSA was 6.6, currently undetectable. Specimen showed Gleason 4 + 3 (Grade Group 2, pT3a, negative margins). He continues with bothersome symptoms of hypogonadism, Total T:267(n = 350–700 ng/dL); Free T:7(n = 9.3–26pg/ml). TTh endorsed with recommendations.

2. A 75 year old with low volume Gleason 3 + 3 (Grade Group 1) CaP on AS. Symptomatic marked hypogonadism leading to TTh. Cumulative moderate increase in PSA with rapid increase 9 years into TTh. T discontinued for 2 years with a subsequent decrease in values. Patient insistent in additional TTh with "excellent grasp" of the issues". Reinitiated TTh with similar results. Patient refused cessation of TTh.

3. A 70-year-old man initially received external beam radiotherapy with 18 months of ADT for high-tier intermediate risk CaP (Grade group 3). PSA nadir at 1.2 ng/mL and steady for 4 years but T never recovered completely (total T: 194 ng/dL). Significant TDS. After extensive shared-decision making process, he decided on TTh with good clinical outcomes and no change in biannual PSA values over 4 years.

CLINICS CARE POINTS

- There is a need for guiding criteria for the general urologist regarding testosterone administration in men with a history of prostate cancer

- Documentation (clinical and biochemical) of hypogonadism is of paramount importance before considering testosterone treatment.
- Strict follow-up is mandatory, particularly in the early stages of testosterone administration.
- Men successfully treated for prostate cancer can safely receive testosterone therapy.
- Hypogonadal men harboring prostate cancer on active surveillance are candidates with specific restrictions.
- Those with intermediate of hig- risk prostate cancer are best managed by specialized centers.
- Participation in clinical trials and registries will help to establish reliable evidence on the safety of testosterone in hypogonadal men.

DISCLOSURE

The authors have nothing to disclose

REFERENCES

1. Thomson WO. Uses and abuses of the male sex hormone. JAMA 1946;132:186–94.
2. Morales A. The long and tortuous history of the discovery of testosterone and its clinical application. J Sex Med 2013;1178–83.
3. Joseph IB, Nelson JB, Denmeade SR, et al. Androgens regulate vascular endothelial growth factor content in normal and malignant prostatic tissue. Clin Cancer Res 1997;3:2507–11.
4. Seeger's MP, Cymene LA, Nadeer AM, et al. How strong is the association between CAG and GGN repeat length polymorphisms in the androgen receptor and prostate cancer risk? Cancer Epidemiol Biomarkers Prep 2004;13:1765–71.
5. Marks LS, Mazer NA, Mustache E, et al. Effect of testosterone replacement therapy on prostate tissue in men with late-onset hypogonadism. JAMA 2006;296:2351–61.
6. Tan MHE, Li J, Xu, et al. Androgen receptor: structure, role in prostate cancer and drug discovery. Act Pharmacol Sin 2015;36:3–23.
7. Yu G, Mylander C, Traish A, et al. Circulating levels of gonadotropins before and after prostate ablation in cancer patients. Horm Mol Biol Clin Invest 2012;11:355–62.
8. Hoare D, Skinner TA, Black A, et al. Serum follicle stimulating hormone levels predict time to development of castration-resistant prostate cancer. Can Urol Assis J 2015;9:122–7.
9. Montgomery RB, Mustache EA, Vesella R, et al. Maintenance of intratumoral androgens in metastatic prostate cancer: a mechanism for castration-resistant tumor growth. Cancer Res 2008;68:4447–54.
10. Haffner MC, Zwart W, Roudier MP, et al. Genomic and phenotypic heterogeneity in prostate cancer. Nat Rev Urol 2021;18:79–92.
11. Das Gupta A, Krawczynska N, Nelson ER. Extracellular vesicles-the next frontier in endocrinology. Endocrinology 2021;162:1–17.
12. Ludwig M, Rajvansh R, Drake JM. Emerging role of extracellular vesicles in prostate cancer. Endocrinology 2021;162:1–10.
13. Pernigoni N, Zagato E, Cacinotto A, et al. Commensal bacteria promote endocrine resistance in prostate cancer. Science 2021;374:216–24.
14. Cackowski FC, Heath EI. Prostate cancer dormancy and recurrence. Cancer Lett 2022;524:103–8.
15. Meeks JJ, Schaeffer EM. Genetic regulation of prostate development. J Androl 2011;32:210–7.
16. Feng Q, He B. Androgen receptor signaling in the development of castration-resistant prostate cancer. Front Oncol 2019. https://doi.org/10.3389/fonc.2019.00858.
17. Davey RA, Grossman M. Androgen receptor structure, function and biology: from bench to bedside. Clin Biochem Rev 2016;37:3–15. PMC4810760 PMID:27057074.
18. Campbell KJ, Leung H. Evasion of cell death: a contributory factor in prostate cancer development and treatment resistance. Cancer Lett 2021;520:213–21.
19. Litvinov IV, De Marzo AM, Isaacs JT. Is the Achilles' heel for prostate cancer therapy a gain of function in androgen receptor signaling? J Clin Endocrinol Metab 2003;88:2972–82.
20. Nelson WG, De Marzo AM, Issacs WB. Mechanisms of Disease: Prostate Cancer. N Engl J Med 2003;349:361–6.
21. Hur J, Giovanucci E. Racial differences in prostate cancer: does timing of puberty play a role. ? Br J Cancer 2020;123:349–54.
22. Thompson IM, Goodman PJ, Tangen CM, et al. The influence of finasteride in the development of prostate cancer. N Engl J Med 2003;349:215–24.
23. Morgentaler A, Bruning CE, DeWolf WC. Occult prostate cancer in men with low serum testosterone levels. JAMA 1996;276:1904–6. PMID 8968017.
24. Morgentaler A, Rhoden EL. Prevalence of prostate cancer among hypogonadal men with prostate-specific antigen level of 4.0ng/mL or less. Urology 2006;68:1263–7.
25. Svatek RS, Schulman MJ, Benaim EA, et al. Change in prostate specific antigen following androgen stimulation is an independent predictor of prostate cancer diagnosis. J Urol 2008;179:2192–5.

26. McKay RR, Xie W, Ye H, et al. Results of a randomized phase II trial of intense androgen deprivation therapy prior to radical prostatectomy in men with high-risk localized prostate cancer. J Urol 2021; 2068:80–7.

27. Shah H, Vaishamppayan U. Therapy of advanced prostate cancer: targeting the androgen receptor axis in earlier lines of treatment. Target Oncol 2018;13:679–89.

28. Loughlin KR, Richie JP. Prostate cancer after exogenous testosterone treatment for impotence. J Urol 1997;157:1845–6.

29. Curran MJ, Bihrle W 3rd. Dramatic rise in PSA after androgen replacement in a hypogonadal man with occult adenocarcinoma of the prostate. Urology 1999;53:423–4.

30. Pierce KM, Miklavcic WR, Cook KP, et al. The evolution and future of targeted cancer therapy: from nanoparticles, oncolytic viruses, and oncolytic bacteria to the treatment of solid tumors. Nanomaterials 2021;11:3018–60.

31. Higgins C. Two principles in endocrine therapy of cancers: hormone deprival and hormone interference. Cancer Res 1965;25:1163–7. PMID: 5897831.

32. Labrie F, Belanger A, Cusan L, et al. Physiological changes in dehydroepiandrosterone are not reflected by serum levels of active androgens and estrogens but their metabolites: intracrinology. J Clin Endocrinol Metab 1997;82:2403–9.

33. Mostaghel EA, Nelson PS. Intracrine androgen metabolism in prostate cancer progression: mechanisms of castration resistance and therapeutic implications. Best Pract Res Clin Endocrinol Metab 2008; 22:243–58.

34. Schiffer L, Arlt W, Storbeck H-H. Intracrine androgen biosynthesis, metabolism and action revisited. *Mol Cell Endocrinol* 2018;465:4–26.

35. Hamid AR, Tendi W, Sesari SS, et al. The importance of targeting intracrinology in prostate cancer management. World J Urol 2019;37:751–7.

36. Morales A, Bebb RA, Manjoo P, et al. Diagnosis and management of testosterone deficiency syndrome in men: clinical practice guideline. CMAJ 2015;187: 1369–78.

37. Mulhall JP, Trost LW, Brannigan RE, et al. Evaluation and management of testosterone deficiency: AUA guideline. J Urol 2018;200:423–32.

38. Bhasin S, Brito JP, Cunningham GR, et al. Testosterone therapy in men with hypogonadism: An Endocrine Society clinical practice guideline. J Clin Endocrinol Metab 2018;1715–44.

39. Chen T, Li S, Eisenberg ML. Trends in testosterone therapy use in prostate cancer survivors in the United States. J Sex Med 2021;18:1346–53.

40. Corona G, Goulis DG, Huhtaniemi I, et al. European Academy of Andrology guidelines on investigation, treatment and monitoring of functional hypogonadism in males. Andrology 2020;8:970–87.

41. Pastuszak AW, Pearlman AM, Lai WS, et al. Testosterone replacement therapy in patients with prostate cancer after radical prostatectomy. J Urol 2013;190: 639–44.

42. Sarkar R, Patel SH, Parsons JK, et al. Testosterone therapy does not increase the risks prostate cancer recurrence or death after definitive treatment for localized disease. Prostate Cancer Prostatic Dis 2020;23:689–95.

43. Sarosdy MF Testosterone replacement for hypogonadism after treatment for early prostate cancer with brachytherapy. Cancer 2007;109:536–41.

44. Morales A, Black AM, Emerson LE. Testosterone administration to men with testosterone deficiency syndrome after external beam radiotherapy for localized prostate cancer: Preliminary observations. BJU Int 2008;103:62–4.

45. Pastuszak AW, Pearlman AM, Godoy G, et al. Testosterone replacement therapy in the setting of prostate cancer treated with radiation. Int J Impotence Res 2013;25:24–8.

46. Ahlering TE, Huynh LM, Towe M, et al. Testosterone replacement therapy reduces biochemical recurrence after radical prostatectomy. BJUI 2020;126: 91–6.

47. Isbar H, Pinthus JH, Marks LS, et al. Testosterone and prostate cancer: revisiting old paradigms. Eur Urol 2009;56:48–56.

48. Morales A. Should hypogonadal men with prostate cancer receive testosterone? – NO. J Urol 2010; 184:1257–60.

49. Mulhall JP, Deveci S, Flores J, et al. Testosterone (T) challenge in men post-radical prostatectomy (RP) with profoundly low testosterone. (Poster.) J Urol 2021;206(Suppl). .) No. 3S. e636.

50. Chen T, Li S, Eisenberg ML. Trends in testosterone therapy use in prostate cancer survivors in the United States. J Sex Med 2021;18:1346–53.

51. Mason MM, Nackeeran S, Lokeshwar SD, et al. PSA testing in men receiving testosterone therapy with history of prostate cancer: a matched analysis of a large multi-institutional research network. Urology 2022. https://doi.org/10.1016/j.urol.2022.02.010.

52. Morgentaler A. Testosterone therapy can be given to me with no concern that it will promote prostate cancer development or progression. J Urol 2016;196: 985–8.

53. Crowley F, Sterpi M, Buckley C, et al. A review of the pathophysiological mechanisms underlying castration-resistant prostate cancer. Res Rep Urol 2021;13:457–72.

54. Chih-pin C, Hiipakka RA, Fukuchi J, et al. Androgens cause growth suppression and reversion of androgen-independent prostate cancer xenografts

to an androgen-stimulated phenotype in athymic mice. Cancer Res 2005;65:2082–4.

55. Hatzoglu A, Kampa M, Kogia C, et al. Membrane androgen receptor activation induces apoptotic regression of human prostate cancer cells in vitro and in vivo. J Clin Endocrinol Metab 2005;90: 893–903.

56. Sanda MG, Chen RC, Crispino T, et al. Clinically localized prostate cancer: AUA/ASTRO/SUO guideline. Available at: www.auanet.org/guidelines/clinically-localized-prostate-cancer-new(aua/astro/suo-guideline-2017).

57. Morales A. Testosterone replacement in a man with intermediate-risk prostate cancer. Eur Urol Focus 2017;319–20.

58. De Sousa A, Sonavane S, Metha J. Psychological aspects of prostate cancer: a clinical review. Prost Cancer Prost Dis 2012;15:120–7.

59. Fervaha G, Izard JP, Tripp DA, et al. Psychological morbidity associated with prostate cancer: rates and predictors of depression in the RADICAL PC study. Can Urol Ass J 2021;15:181–6.

60. Kawakami J, Morales A. Clinical significance of suboptimal hormonal levels in men with prostate cancer treated with LHRH agonists. Can Urol Ass J 2013;7: 226–30.

61. Morales A. Effect of testosterone administration to men with prostate cancer is unpredictable: a word of caution and suggestions for a registry. BJUI 2011;107:1369–73.

62. Pastuszak AW, Pearlman AM, Lai WS, et al. Testosterone replacement therapy in patients with prostate cancer after radical prostatectomy. J Urol 2013;190: 639–44.

63. Balbontin FG, Moreno SA, Bley E, et al. Long-acting testosterone injections for treatment of testosterone deficiency after brachytherapy for prostate cancer. BJU Int 2014;114:125–30.

64. Feltquate D, Nordquist L, Eicher C, et al. Rapid androgen cycling as treatment for patients with cancer. Clin Cancer Res 2006;12:7414–21.

65. Schwitzer MT, Antonarakis ES, Wan H, et al. Effect of bipolar androgen therapy for asymptomatic men with castration-resistant prostate cancer: Results from a pilot clinical study. Sci Transl Med 2015;7: 269–72.

66. Denmeade SR, Isaacs JT. Bipolar androgen therapy: the rationale for rapid cycling of supraphysiological androgen/ablation in men with castration resistant prostate cancer. Prostate 2010;70:1600–7.

67. Sena LA, Wang H, Lim SJ, et al. Bipolar androgen therapy sensitizes castration-resistant prostate cancer to subsequent androgen receptors ablative therapy. Eur J Cancer 2021;144:302–9.

68. Denmeade SR, Wang H, Agarwal N, et al. TRANSFORMER: A randomized phase II study comparing bipolar androgen therapy versus enzalutamide in asymptomatic men with castration-resistant metastatic prostate cancer. J Clin Oncol 2021;39: 1371–82.

69. Clinical Trials.gov Bipolar Androgen therapy (BAT) and radium-223 (RAD) in metastatic-castration resistant prostate cancer (mCRPC) (BAT-RAD) Clinical trials identifier: NCT04704505.

70. Morgentaler A. Testosterone therapy can be given to men with no concern that it will promote prostate cancer development or progression. J Urol 2016; 196:985–7.

71. Morales A, Connolly JG, Bruce AW. Androgen therapy in advanced carcinoma of the prostate. Can Med Assoc J 1971;105:71–3.

72. Fowler JE Jr, Whitmore WF Jr. The response of metastatic adenocarcinoma of the prostate to exogenous testosterone. J Urol 1981;126:372–5.

73. Morales A. Effect of testosterone administration to men with prostate cancer is unpredictable: a word of caution and suggestions for a registry. BJUI 2011;107:1369–73.

74. Isbar H, Pinthus JH, Marks LS, et al. Testosterone and prostate cancer: revisiting old paradigms. Eur Urol 2009;56:48–56.

75. Morgentaler A, Traish A. Shifting the paradigm of testosterone and prostate cancer: the saturation model and the limits of androgen dependent growth. Eur Urol 2009;55:310–20.

76. Kraker R, Hult M, Sanfrancisco IF, et al. Can testosterone therapy be offered to men on active surveillance for prostate cancer? Preliminary results. Asian J. Androl 2016;18:16–20.

77. Morgentaler A, Lipshultz BR, Bennett R, et al. Testosterone therapy in men with untreated prostate cancer. J Urol 2011;185:1256–60.

78. Shoag J, Barbieri CE. Clinical variability and molecular heterogeneity in prostate cancer. Asian J Androl 2016;18:543–8.

79. Lakshman KM, Kaplan B, Travison TG, et al. The effects of injected testosterone dose and age on the conversion of testosterone to estradiol and dihydrotestosterone in young and older men. J Clin Endocrinol Metab 2010;95:3955–64.

80. Goldenberg L, So A, Fleshner N, et al. The role of 5-alpha reductase inhibitors in prostate pathophysiology: is there and additional advantage to inhibition of type 1 isoenzyme? Can Urol Ass J 2009;(OSuppl 2):S109–14.

81. Kim JW. Questioning the evidence behind the saturation model for testosterone replacement therapy in prostate cancer. Investig Clin Urol 2020;61:242–9.

82. Kim M, Byun S-S, Hong SK. Testosterone replacement therapy in men with untreated or treated prostate cancer: Do we have enough evidence? World J Mens Health 2021;39:705–23.

83. Gleave ME, Klotz L. Testosterone therapy can be given to men with no concern that it will promote

prostate cancer development or progression. J Urol 2016;196:985.

84. Michaud JE, Billups KL, Partin AW. Testosterone and prostate cancer: an evidence-based review of pathogenesis and oncologic risk. Ther Adv Urol 2015;7: 378–87.

85. Nguyen TM, Pastuszak AW. Testosterone therapy among prostate cancer survivors. Sex Med Rev 2016;4:376388.

86. Pastuszak AW, Rodriguez KM, Nguyen TM, et al. Testosterone therapy and prostate cancer. Transl Androl Urol 2016;5:909–20.

87. Kim M, Byun S-S, Hong SK. Testosterone replacement therapy in men with untreated or treated prostate cancer: Do we have enough evidence? World J Men's Health 2021;39:705–23.

88. Bhasin S, Singh AB, Mac RP, et al. Managing the risks of prostate disease during testosterone replacement therapy in older men: recommendations for a standardized monitoring plan. Andrology 2003;24:299–311.

89. Araujo AB, O'Donell Ab, Brambilla DJ, et al. Prevalence and incidence of androgen deficiency in middle-aged and older men: estimates from the Massachusetts Male Aging Study. J Clin Endocrin Metab 2004;89:5920.

90. Cooperberg MR, Broering JM, Litwin MS, et al. The contemporary management of prostate cancer in the United States: lessons from the cancer of the prostate strategic urological research endeavor (CapSURE), a national disease registry. J Urol 2004;171:1393–401.

91. Sayyid RK, Klotz L, Benton JZ, et al. Active surveillance in favorable intermediate-risk prostate cancer patients: predictor of deferred intervention and treatment choice. CUAJ 2022;16:E7–14.

92. Leapman MS, Wang R, Park HS, et al. Adoption of new risk stratification technologies within US hospital referral regions and association with prostatic cancer management. JAMA Netw Open 2021; 4(10):e2128646.

93. Clark R, Kenk M, McAlpine K, et al. The evolving role of germline genetic testing and management in prostate cancer: report from the Princess Margaret Cancer Centre international retreat. Can Urol Assoc J 2021;15:623–9.

94. Russo J, McDougall C, Bowler N, et al. Pretest genetic education video versus genetic counseling for men considering prostate cancer germline testing: a patient-choice study to address urgent practice needs. JCO Precis Oncol 2021;5:1377–86.

95. NG TSC, Gao X, Salari K, et al. Incorporating PSMA-targeting theranostics into personalized prostate cancer treatment: a multidisciplinary perspective. Front Oncol 2021;11:722277.

96. Wallis CJD, Zhao Z, Huang L-C, et al. Association of treatment modality, functional outcomes, and baseline characteristics with treatment-related regret among men with localized prostate cancer. JAMA Oncol 2021. https://doi.org/10.1001/jamaoncol.2021.5160.

Current Management and Controversies Surrounding Andropause

Abrar H. Mian, BS[a], David Y. Yang, MD[b], Tobias S. Kohler, MD, MPH[c,*]

KEYWORDS

- Testosterone • Hypogonadism • Andropause • TRT

KEY POINTS

- Although the treatment of hypogonadism is dependent on symptoms and symptom improvement, total testosterone, along with free testosterone and sex hormone-binding globulin, should be considered when correctly diagnosing a patient.
- Testosterone therapy is not without potential side effects. Physician's oversight is critical to optimize outcomes and minimize risk.
- Although testosterone replacement therapy is not indicated to treat obesity, diabetes, or complications of a sedentary lifestyle, diagnosis and treatment of concomitant hypogonadism may facilitate a healthier lifestyle.

INTRODUCTION

Andropause is defined by a decrease in serum testosterone below the normal range accompanied by clinical symptoms, such as lethargy, decreased libido, concentration issues, depression, decreased sleep, and so forth. The Massachusetts Male Aging Study estimated that approximately 2.4 million 40 to 69-year-old men in the United States have androgen deficiency (AD) and concluded that the rate increased significantly with age.[1] Additionally, 35% of men in their 70s have been shown to have lower testosterone levels than younger men.[2] Between 1959 and 2016, life expectancy in the United States increased by nearly a decade.[3] These realities show that andropause deserves more attention and awareness, as it becomes more prevalent.

Definitions and Pathophysiology

Hypogonadism, according to the American Urologic Association (AUA), refers to males who have serum testosterone less than 300 ng/dL, as confirmed by two tests in the morning along with pertinent symptoms.[4] There are several mechanisms in which this condition can manifest, as denoted by the specific classifications. Primary hypogonadism presents with decreased testosterone and elevated gonadotropin levels because of underlying testicular failure. Secondary hypogonadism presents with both a decreased serum testosterone and decreased gonadotropin levels because of underlying pathology of the hypothalamic–pituitary axis. For cases where testosterone production is impaired but gonadotropin levels remain within the normal range, the Sexual Medicine Society of North America developed a diagnosis termed adult-onset hypogonadism. Adult-onset hypogonadism presents with the same symptoms as hypogonadism and is acquired in adulthood.[5]

Hypogonadism can still manifest without underlying pathology due to old age, in a condition called late-onset hypogonadism or andropause.

[a] Midwestern University, Chicago College of Osteopathic Medicine, 555 31st Street, Downers Grove, IL 60515, USA; [b] Department of Urology, Emory University, 100 Woodruff Circle, Atlanta, GA 30322, USA; [c] Department of Urology, Mayo Clinic: Rochester, 200 First Street Southwest, Rochester, MN 55905, USA
* Corresponding author.
E-mail address: kohler.tobias@mayo.edu
Twitter: @AbrarMian8 (A.H.M.); @YangUrology (D.Y.Y.); @SexHealthMD (T.S.K.)

Urol Clin N Am 49 (2022) 583–592
https://doi.org/10.1016/j.ucl.2022.07.003
0094-0143/22/© 2022 Elsevier Inc. All rights reserved.

Late-onset hypogonadism is characterized by the combination of signs and symptoms suggestive of AD and consistently low serum testosterone levels for no apparent reason other than age itself.[6] The European Male Aging Study surveyed 3369 men aged 40 to 79 years and found that the prevalence of late-onset hypogonadism in their population was 2.1% and would increase with age from 0.1% for men 40 to 49 years of age, to 0.6% for those 50 to 59 years, to 3.2% for those 60 to 69 years, and to 5.1% for those 70 to 79 years. They found late-onset hypogonadism to be associated with at least three sexual symptoms (decreased sexual thoughts, erectile dysfunction, and weakened morning erections) and a total testosterone level of less than 317 ng/dL (11 nmol/L) and a free testosterone level of less than 17 ng/dL (220 pmol per liter).[7]

Current Management and Modalities

Before starting testosterone replacement therapy (TRT), patients should be tested to ensure they are in fact testosterone deficient. Even further, it is important to constantly monitor the testosterone level in these individuals to ensure the patient's testosterone falls within the target range, with the AUA denoting between 450 and 600 ng/dL.[4] These points are imperative, as it is reported that nearly a third of men placed on TRT do not actually qualify as testosterone-deficient.[8] Malik and colleagues reported that in 3320 hypogonadal men receiving TRT, 49% did not have follow-up checkups.[9] The current AUA guidelines indicate that a testosterone level below 300 ng/dL achieved after two measurements taken on separate occasions early in the morning classifies as testosterone-deficient. Additionally, measuring luteinizing hormone levels may aid in determining the etiology of the deficiency.[4] Once the diagnosis of hypogonadism is confirmed, testosterone treatment can be conducted while being closely monitored for 3, 6, and 12 months, and then annually. In addition to testing their serum testosterone levels, patients should also be interviewed for physical and mental activity, libido, and sexual activity.[10] Of all the modalities available for measuring serum testosterone, gas or liquid chromatography-tandem mass spectrometry offers the least amount of variability when compared with immunoassays.[11]

In treating hypogonadism, there are a variety of treatment options, with TRT being the primary option. There are several means of administration, such as oral, intramuscular injections, transdermal patches/gels/pumps/solutions, subdermal implants, and nasal applications.[12] In a situation where testosterone treatment is contraindicated or the patient wishes to avert its side effects (ie, infertility) there are alternative options available, such as human chorionic gonadotropin, aromatase inhibitors, selective estrogen receptor modulators, or implementation of lifestyle changes.[13] Several factors play a role in deciding which form is best for the patient, such as ease of application, patient abuse potential, and expense. In this review, we focus on several of the modern controversies associated with TRT.

DISCUSSION
Making the Diagnosis

Many official guidelines in place today, such as the AUA, diagnose someone as testosterone-deficient by looking at their serum total testosterone levels. Even within these guidelines; however, there is still ambiguity. If a patient presents with low-normal testosterone levels but displays symptoms of hypogonadism, are their symptoms justified for TRT? What about the patients who are receiving TRT because they met the guidelines, and although their levels improve, their symptoms persist? In both cases, looking at total testosterone concentrations as the sole serum marker provides an incomplete picture at times. Antonio and colleagues found that men with normal total testosterone but low free testosterone demonstrated the highest proportion of men with infrequent sexual thought, erectile dysfunction, and infrequent morning erections, whereas these sexual symptoms were not observed in men with low total testosterone and normal free testosterone.[14] Sex hormone binding globulin (SHBG) may also play a role in a more accurate diagnosis of hypogonadism. Ring and colleagues found that only 49% of the patients with total testosterone greater than 300 ng/dL could be considered eugonadal in light of their calculated bioavailable testosterone. Additionally, for patients that had total testosterone below 300 ng/dL, 19% of them could be considered eugonadal by calculating their bioavailable levels. In both instances, using SHBG levels to calculate the free testosterone levels provided further insight into the patient's diagnosis.[15] Although guidelines recommend diagnosing hypogonadism based on serum total testosterone levels, they may misdiagnose and undertreat a substantial number of patients. In a patient with low-normal total testosterone, free testosterone levels and SHBG may be used to further diagnose the symptomatic patient (**Fig. 1** [free testosterone value in figure approximated from European guidelines]).[16]

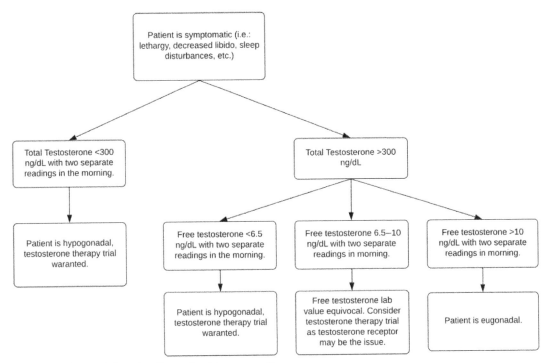

Fig. 1. Flowchart guiding the diagnosis of hypogonadism.

It is imperative to acknowledge that the most important outcome of TRT is whether the patient has symptom improvement. Questions, such as whether the patient is feeling symptomatic improvement or able to implement healthier habits due to the therapy, should be asked. If a patient is receiving therapy and his/her total testosterone levels fall within the target range of 450 to 600 ng/dL for 3 months, but he/she still does not feel a difference, we recommend the "stop and start" approach. Cease TRT with the patient for a period of time and observe how they react. Naturally, their serum testosterone levels will sharply decrease because of the effects of negative feedback from the exogenous testosterone, resulting in atrophy of the hormonal gland. Once their levels return to what they were before TRT, however, ask the patients if they notice a difference. If they are feeling worse, restart testosterone replacement and continue to monitor the patient. Additional factors that must be considered are whether the patient has an underlying condition (ie, human immunodeficiency virus) that results in the deviation of their SHBG level. Symptomatic patients may have an abnormally high serum total testosterone, but if their bioavailable testosterone is minimal, they will be hypogonadal.

Testosterone Therapy and Misinformation

Baillargeon and colleagues reported that from 2001 to 2011, androgen use in men 40 years or older had increased threefold, and that among all new users in that time frame, 25% had not had their levels measured the prior year.[17] This trend of testosterone being prescribed in men not meeting guidelines is worrisome, and may in large part have to do with misinformation and advertising. Warren and colleagues recently published a study looking at how many people depend on YouTube as a means of TRT information. The 80 videos analyzed amassed a total of 38,549,090 views. A concerning finding was that the videos created by nonphysicians and harbored misinformation had significantly more views than those featuring physicians.[18] Other contributing factors toward increased off-labeled use include aggressive direct-to-consumer marketing for low testosterone treatment, the establishment of clinics dedicated to prescribing testosterone, Internet pharmacies in Canada with sales in the United States, and the availability of new transdermal testosterone preparations, which increase the ease of use.[19] Ambiguity of guidelines also play a part in this phenomenon.[20] Although efforts toward amending these discrepancies are being made, a greater push must be taken. In combatting misinformation, accredited experts should work to provide reliable content in a more accessible and understandable manner.

Testosterone Therapy and Cardiovascular Disease

The risk of cardiovascular disease (CVD) in association with TRT has been a controversial topic. Early studies looking at TRT and CVD found a positive correlation between TRT use and adverse cardiac outcomes. One retrospective study evaluating hypogonadal men on TRT found that within 3 years, 25.7% of the group receiving TRT experienced adverse cardiac events compared with the 19.9% who had not received therapy.[21] Another retrospective study came to a similar conclusion, claiming that in men with pre-existing heart disease, those receiving TRT had a substantially greater risk of experiencing a myocardial infarction.[22] In 2016, a board of experts convened and stated that both of these studies were critically flawed and that there is great evidence demonstrating there is no correlative risk, yet the FDA still maintains its stance.[23,24] The RHYME (Registry of Hypogonadism in Men) was a large study looking at the potential risk of TRT leading to cardiovascular events in hypogonadal men. The study concluded when controlling for age and before CVD diagnosis, TRT was not a risk factor.[25] This finding has been corroborated by subsequent studies.[26,27]

While the debate regarding TRT in CVD patients continues, there is strong evidence that hypogonadism itself is a risk factor for CVD. Araujo and colleagues performed a meta-analysis investigating hypogonadism and CD. They found low testosterone to be significantly associated with all-cause mortality and strongly associated, although not statistically significant, with cardiovascular mortality.[28] Another meta-analysis conducted by Corona and colleagues found that lower testosterone and higher estradiol levels were significantly associated with an increased risk of CVD.[29] Because of these findings, the AUA guidelines recommend educating patients on the association between low testosterone and CVD. As such, TRT, when appropriately monitored, should be offered to patients with CVD, but TRT should not be initiated within 3 to 6 months following a cardiovascular event.[4]

Testosterone Therapy and the Prostate

For the greater part of the past century, it has been postulated that TRT stimulates prostate cancer and castration reduces metastatic cancers.[30,31]

As such, an active or history of prostate cancer was a contraindication for TRT. More recently, this notion has been challenged. In 2009, Morgentaler and Traish[32] published their work on their saturation model for the androgen receptor. They found that testosterone levels above the "saturation point" (well below the physiologically normal concentration) would have little to no effect on prostate growth. Alternatively, providing testosterone to castrated patients will result in prostate growth as their physiologic testosterone concentration is below the saturation point.[32] As such, TRT in the appropriately counseled and monitored patient can be considered. To further cloud our understanding of testosterone and prostate cancer, Schweizer and colleagues observed that the use of super-physiologic levels of testosterone suppressed some advanced prostate cancers and may also have the potential to reverse the resistance to testosterone-blocking drugs used to treat prostate cancer.[33] While much larger scale, prospective analyses are needed to derive substantial proof, these studies demonstrate that there is much more nuance to this subject and provides a greater perspective on how TRT and prostate cancer are viewed.

In regard to the effect TRT has on benign prostatic hyperplasia (BPH) and lower urinary tract symptoms; despite a prevalent notion that there is an increased risk of symptom exacerbation, an in-depth literature review concluded hypogonadism was itself a risk factor for these symptoms, and that TRT improved BPH symptoms.[34] Despite this evidence, testosterone products, such as AndroGel, caution physicians about the risk of BPH development and also cite prostatic disorders as an adverse reaction.[35] Labels, such as this, deter physicians from initiating TRT in hypogonadal patients that may benefit from it, and so it is imperative for physicians to be aware of what the literature states on this subject and counsel patients accordingly.

Testosterone Therapy and Thrombosis

It is known that TRT has been linked with an increased incidence of polycythemia.[36,37] In regard to whether TRT is a risk factor for distal venous thrombosis, retrospective studies have found it is not.[38,39] Glueck and colleagues reviewed 596 patients hospitalized with thrombosis, the few patients that were on exogenous testosterone were ultimately found to have an undiagnosed hypercoagulability abnormality.[40] They conducted a similar study investigating men with Klinefelter syndrome and saw once again that only those with a prothrombotic condition went on to develop thrombosis.[41] Although larger studies are needed to corroborate these findings, screening men for prothrombotic conditions before initiating TRT is recommended. Ory and colleagues evaluated the association of TRT-induced polycythemia with thrombotic events. After matching for 14 risk factors, they found patients with TRT-induced polycythemia were at an increased risk of acute myocardial infarction or venous thromboembolic events. The risk of developing a stroke or death, however, was similar between the two groups.[42]

Testosterone Therapy and Therapeutic Phlebotomies

Therapeutic phlebotomy along with changing testosterone dosing or formulation is the mainstay in combatting TRT-induced polycythemia. A study conducted by Van Buren and colleagues investigated the incidence of men on TRT seeking phlebotomies. They noted that between 2014 and 2016, on average, patients on TRT received 2.8 to 3.8 therapeutic phlebotomies per year. A retrospective review of their data noted that 32% of patients who previously received phlebotomy returned to their center to donate blood, as a means of receiving a "free phlebotomy."[43] Similarly, Hazegh and colleagues found that men on TRT visited donation centers much more frequently than men not on TRT.[44] Although voluntary blood donation may be a convenient option for patients, Peeden and colleagues highlight the benefits of therapeutic phlebotomy. Not only is the patient able to receive higher volumes of phlebotomy than normally permitted for a "healthy" blood donor, but it also facilitates communication and appropriate monitoring between the patient and provider.[45]

Testosterone Therapy and Antiaging Effects

As men age, there is a gradual decline seen in their testosterone levels, and it is thought that many of the age-related functional declines may be linked to hypogonadism. The testosterone trials investigated the effects of TRT on seven different trial groups in hypogonadal men greater than 65 years of age. The sexual function trial, physical function trial, and vitality trial demonstrated statistically significant improvement in outcome measures. The cognitive function trial showed no improvement in any cognitive tests. The anemia trial showed improved hemoglobin in low testosterone, anemic men. The bone trial displayed an impressive increase in volumetric bone marrow density and estimated bone strength. This improvement was noted to be at least as much as the effect of

bisphosphonates on volumetric bone marrow density in women with osteoporosis. The cardiovascular trial saw that the treatment group had an increase in noncalcified coronary artery plaque volume, but longer and larger trials needed to be performed to see if this finding correlated to increased clinical cardiovascular risk. Although the treatment group showed an increase in PSA, it could not be concluded that TRT correlated to an increased risk of prostate cancer.[46]

Exogenous Testosterone Abuse

The use of exogenous testosterone as a performance-enhancing drug has been a growing trend in a large part due to its performance-enhancing abilities, quick effect, along with the gradual reform of the Western cultural view on male masculinity.[47] While the majority of anabolic, adrenergic steroid (AAS) use is seen mostly in individuals under the age of 60,[48] its relevance in this discussion is especially important as this cohort will be the basis of observing the long-term effects of AAS abuse in the aging population. Currently, it is known that exogenous steroid abuse (beyond super therapeutic levels) results in many cardiac side effects, such as hypertension, dyslipidemia, cardiomyopathy, left ventricular hypertrophy, myocardial ischemia, and arrhythmia.[49–60] Psychiatric side effects include aggressiveness, exaggerated self-confidence, hyperactivity, reckless behavior irritability, and occasional psychotic symptoms.[61–63] Depressive symptoms were also noted, such as loss of interest, loss of libido, anorexia, and sometimes suicidal ideation.[64–66] A plethora of other side effects exist, such as testicular atrophy, erectile dysfunction, gynecomastia, and others.[67] A concerning finding was that nearly 56% of patient AAS users revealed through a survey that they do not disclose their AAS use with their physicians.[68] This subject is extremely relevant because of the potential downstream effects on an aging population.

Testosterone Therapy and Type 2 Diabetes Mellitus

The controversy regarding the use of TRT to prevent the progression of type 2 diabetes mellitus (T2DM) is in large part due to the staunch guidelines in place regarding TRT and the many discussed side effects. Low levels of total testosterone and free testosterone have been shown to be independent predictive factors for the development of T2DM.[69–74] Patients are often told to lose weight and implement better lifestyle habits, a tall task for a hypogonadal patient. This approach sets unrealistic expectations for patients, and its ineffectiveness can be seen with the increasing prevalence of this condition.[75] The BLAST study investigated the effects of testosterone undecanoate in achieving serum testosterone levels in patients with T2DM. Patients were categorized into two groups based on testosterone levels (MILD and SEVERE) and received long-acting testosterone undecanoate for 30 weeks, followed by open-label use for 52 weeks. Men in the MILD group saw significant improvement in weight, body mass index, waist circumference, and decline in depressive symptoms. The SEVERE group did not see significant improvement in these areas but had an impressive improvement in sexual function.[76] A large-scale, double-blind, randomized, placebo-controlled Australian-based study looked at the role of testosterone treatment in preventing or reversing T2DM in men enrolled in a lifestyle program. They found that patients receiving testosterone had a decreased incidence of T2DM compared with those in the placebo group. Although TRT is not indicated to treat T2DM, screening for hypogonadism should be considered to help facilitate lifestyle changes.[77]

SUMMARY

TRT has been an area of great controversy in the aging male population. On one end, treatment may be administered loosely without monitoring, and on the other extreme, it is seen as a taboo prescription. As we see an increase in men living longer and manifesting symptoms of andropause, it is the role of the physician to be informed about the appropriate role of TRT. This entails the physician having a conversation with his/her patient about the realistic risks and benefits of treatment. In this review, we hope that addressing modern-day controversies associated with TRT in a simple, practical way will help physicians become more familiar with the nuances surrounding it, and provide their patients with the best possible care.

CLINICS CARE POINTS

Controversies	Key Points
Diagnosing hypogonadism	• Free testosterone levels should be calculated if a symptomatic patient has a total testosterone >300 ng/dL.

Controversies	Key Points
	• Patients should be treated as individuals and priority should be given to how they are responding to treatment as opposed to laboratory values. Guidelines help approximate treatment, but individuals may respond differently to different levels.
Misinformation	• YouTube videos from nonexperts receive many more views than videos from experts discussing TRT.
• Many factors facilitate the unregulated administration of testosterone, such as aggressive marketing, testosterone-specific clinics, and products that are easy to use (ie, transdermal patches).
Cardiovascular disease	• TRT is not a risk factor for CVD.
• Low testosterone is actually a risk factor for CVD.
• TRT should not be initiated within 3–6 mo of a cardiovascular event.
The prostate	• TRT does not increase the risk for prostate cancer.
• Testosterone may have a protective effect against the development of high grade prostate cancers.
• TRT does not increase the risk of developing benign prostatic hyperplasia or lower urinary tract symptoms. In fact, it may help improve them.

(continued on next page)

Controversies	Key Points
Thrombosis	• There may be an increased risk of developing DVTs with TRT-induced polycythemia. • Patients should be screened for potential undiagnosed thrombophilia disorders.
Therapeutic phlebotomies	• There is an increased use of blood donation outside the scope of medical follow-up and clinicians should be overseeing these practices in their patients.
Testosterone trials investigating Antiaging effects	• Improvement seen in sexual function, anemia, and bone strength. • Small improvement seen in physical function and vitality. • No improvement seen in cognitive function.
Exogenous testosterone abuse	• This area has been a growing trend in the past few decades. • 56% of patients in this population admit to not disclosing their steroid use with physicians. • For the first time, we will be witnessing the long-term effects of testosterone abuse in the elderly population.
Type 2 diabetes mellitus	• Low levels of total testosterone and free testosterone have also been shown to be independent predictive factors for development of T2DM. • TRT in these patients helps them implement healthier life styles, improving

Controversies	Key Points
	their overall health and condition.

DISCLOSURE

The authors have nothing to disclose.

REFERENCES

1. Araujo AB, O'Donnell AB, Brambilla DJ, et al. Prevalence and incidence of androgen deficiency in middle-aged and older men: estimates from the Massachusetts Male Aging Study. J Clin Endocrinol Metab 2004;89(12):5920–6.
2. Vermeulen A, Kaufman JM. Ageing of the hypothalamo-pituitary-testicular axis in men. Horm Res 1995;43(1–3):25–8.
3. Woolf SH, Schoomaker H. Life Expectancy and Mortality Rates in the United States, 1959-2017. JAMA 2019;322(20):1996–2016.
4. Mulhall JP, Trost LW, Brannigan RE, et al. Evaluation and Management of Testosterone Deficiency: AUA Guideline. J Urol 2018;200(2):423–32.
5. Khera M, Broderick GA, Carson CC 3rd, et al. Adult-Onset Hypogonadism. Mayo Clin Proc 2016;91(7):908–26.
6. Wang C, Nieschlag E, Swerdloff R, et al. EAA and ASA recommendations: investigation, treatment and monitoring of late-onset hypogonadism in males. Int J Impot Res b 2009;21(1):1–8.
7. Wu FC, Tajar A, Beynon JM, et al. Identification of late-onset hypogonadism in middle-aged and elderly men. N Engl J Med 2010;363(2):123–35.
8. Baillargeon J, Urban RJ, Kuo YF, et al. Screening and monitoring in men prescribed testosterone therapy in the U.S., 2001-2010. Public Health Rep 2015;130(2):143–52.
9. Malik RD, Wang CE, Lapin B, et al. Characteristics of Men Undergoing Testosterone Replacement Therapy and Adherence to Follow-up Recommendations in Metropolitan Multicenter Health Care System. Urology 2015;85(6):1382–8.
10. Nieschlag E. Current topics in testosterone replacement of hypogonadal men. Best Pract Res Clin Endocrinol Metab 2015;29(1):77–90.
11. Vesper HW, Bhasin S, Wang C, et al. Interlaboratory comparison study of serum total testosterone [corrected] measurements performed by mass spectrometry methods. Steroids 2009;74(6):498–503.
12. Qaseem A, Horwitch CA, Vijan S, et al. Testosterone Treatment in Adult Men With Age-Related Low Testosterone: A Clinical Guideline From the

American College of Physicians. Ann Intern Med 2020;172(2):126–33.

13. Lo EM, Rodriguez KM, Pastuszak AW, et al. Alternatives to Testosterone Therapy: A Review. Sex Med Rev 2018;6(1):106–13.

14. Antonio L, Wu FC, O'Neill TW, et al. Low Free Testosterone Is Associated with Hypogonadal Signs and Symptoms in Men with Normal Total Testosterone. J Clin Endocrinol Metab 2016;101(7):2647–57.

15. Ring J, Welliver C, Parenteau M, et al. The Utility of Sex Hormone-Binding Globulin in Hypogonadism and Infertile Males. J Urol 2017;197(5):1326–31.

16. Salonia A, Bettocchi C, Boeri L, et al. European Association of Urology Guidelines on Sexual and Reproductive Health-2021 Update: Male Sexual Dysfunction. Eur Urol 2021;80(3):333–57.

17. Baillargeon J, Urban RJ, Ottenbacher KJ, et al. Trends in androgen prescribing in the United States, 2001 to 2011. JAMA Intern Med 2013;173(15): 1465–6.

18. Warren CJ, Wisener J, Ward B, et al. YouTube as a Patient Education Resource for Male Hypogonadism and Testosterone Therapy. Sex Med 2021;9(2): 100324.

19. Jasuja GK, Bhasin S, Rose AJ. Patterns of testosterone prescription overuse. Curr Opin Endocrinol Diabetes Obes 2017;24(3):240–5.

20. Mascarenhas A, Khan S, Sayal R, et al. Factors that may be influencing the rise in prescription testosterone replacement therapy in adult men: a qualitative study. Aging Male 2016;19(2):90–5.

21. Vigen R, O'Donnell CI, Baron AE, et al. Association of testosterone therapy with mortality, myocardial infarction, and stroke in men with low testosterone levels. JAMA 2013;310(17):1829–36.

22. Finkle WD, Greenland S, Ridgeway GK, et al. Increased risk of non-fatal myocardial infarction following testosterone therapy prescription in men. PLoS One 2014;9(1):e85805.

23. Morgentaler A, Zitzmann M, Traish AM, et al. Fundamental Concepts Regarding Testosterone Deficiency and Treatment: International Expert Consensus Resolutions. Mayo Clin Proc 2016; 91(7):881–96.

24. Elagizi A, Kohler TS, Lavie CJ. Testosterone and Cardiovascular Health. Mayo Clin Proc 2018;93(1): 83–100.

25. Maggi M, Wu FC, Jones TH, et al. Testosterone treatment is not associated with increased risk of adverse cardiovascular events: results from the Registry of Hypogonadism in Men (RHYME). Int J Clin Pract 2016;70(10):843–52.

26. Haddad RM, Kennedy CC, Caples SM, et al. Testosterone and cardiovascular risk in men: a systematic review and meta-analysis of randomized placebo-controlled trials. Mayo Clin Proc 2007; 82(1):29–39.

27. Carson CC 3rd, Rosano G. Exogenous testosterone, cardiovascular events, and cardiovascular risk factors in elderly men: a review of trial data. J Sex Med 2012;9(1):54–67.

28. Araujo AB, Dixon JM, Suarez EA, et al. Clinical review: Endogenous testosterone and mortality in men: a systematic review and meta-analysis. J Clin Endocrinol Metab 2011;96(10):3007–19.

29. Corona G, Rastrelli G, Monami M, et al. Hypogonadism as a risk factor for cardiovascular mortality in men: a meta-analytic study. Eur J Endocrinol 2011; 165(5):687–701.

30. Huggins C, Hodges CV. Studies on prostatic cancer. I. The effect of castration, of estrogen and androgen injection on serum phosphatases in metastatic carcinoma of the prostate. CA Cancer J Clin 1972; 22(4):232–40.

31. Fowler JE Jr, Whitmore WF Jr. The response of metastatic adenocarcinoma of the prostate to exogenous testosterone. J Urol 1981;126(3):372–5.

32. Morgentaler A, Traish AM. Shifting the paradigm of testosterone and prostate cancer: the saturation model and the limits of androgen-dependent growth. Eur Urol 2009;55(2):310–20.

33. Schweizer MT, Antonarakis ES, Wang H, et al. Effect of bipolar androgen therapy for asymptomatic men with castration-resistant prostate cancer: results from a pilot clinical study. Sci Transl Med 2015; 7(269):269ra2.

34. Baas W, Kohler TS. Testosterone Replacement Therapy and BPH/LUTS. What is the Evidence? Curr Urol Rep 2016;17(6):46.

35. Reference ID: 3311548 - Food and drug administration.

36. Wald M, Meacham RB, Ross LS, et al. Testosterone replacement therapy for older men. J Androl 2006; 27(2):126–32.

37. Bhasin S, Basaria S. Diagnosis and treatment of hypogonadism in men. Best Pract Res Clin Endocrinol Metab 2011;25(2):251–70.

38. Kavoussi PK, Machen GL, Wenzel JL, et al. Medical Treatments for Hypogonadism do not Significantly Increase the Risk of Deep Vein Thrombosis Over General Population Risk. Urology 2019;124:127–30.

39. Ramasamy R, Scovell J, Mederos M, et al. Association Between Testosterone Supplementation Therapy and Thrombotic Events in Elderly Men. Urology 2015;86(2):283–5.

40. Glueck CJ, Richardson-Royer C, Schultz R, et al. Testosterone therapy, thrombophilia-hypofibrinolysis, and hospitalization for deep venous thrombosis-pulmonary embolus: an exploratory, hypothesis-generating study. Clin Appl Thromb Hemostr 2014;20(3):244–9.

41. Glueck CJ, Jetty V, Goldenberg N, et al. Thrombophilia in Klinefelter Syndrome With Deep Venous Thrombosis, Pulmonary Embolism, and Mesenteric

Artery Thrombosis on Testosterone Therapy: A Pilot Study. Clin Appl Thromb Hemost 2017;23(8):973–9.

42. Ory J, Nackeeran S, Balaji NC, et al. Secondary Polycythemia in Men Receiving Testosterone Therapy Increases Risk of Major Adverse Cardiovascular Events and Venous Thromboembolism in the First Year of Therapy. J Urol 2022;207(6):1295–301, 101097JU0000000000002437.

43. Van Buren NL, Hove AJ, French TA, et al. Therapeutic Phlebotomy for Testosterone-Induced Polycythemia. Am J Clin Pathol 2020;154(1):33–7.

44. Hazegh K, Bravo MD, Kamel H, et al. The prevalence and demographic determinants of blood donors receiving testosterone replacement therapy at a large USA blood service organization. Transfusion 2020;60(5):947–54.

45. Peedin AR, Karp JK. How do I...perform therapeutic phlebotomy? Transfusion 2021;61(3):673–7.

46. Snyder PJ, Bhasin S, Cunningham GR, et al. Lessons From the Testosterone Trials. Endocr Rev 2018;39(3):369–86.

47. Pope H, Phillips KA, Olivardia R. The Adonis complex : the secret crisis of male body obsession, xv. Free Press; 2000. p. 286.

48. Kanayama G, Hudson JI, Pope HG Jr. Long-term psychiatric and medical consequences of anabolic-androgenic steroid abuse: a looming public health concern? Drug Alcohol Depend 2008; 98(1–2):1–12.

49. Urhausen A, Albers T, Kindermann W. Are the cardiac effects of anabolic steroid abuse in strength athletes reversible? Heart 2004;90(5):496–501.

50. Kuipers H, Wijnen JA, Hartgens F, et al. Influence of anabolic steroids on body composition, blood pressure, lipid profile and liver functions in body builders. Int J Sports Med 1991;12(4):413–8.

51. Bonetti A, Tirelli F, Catapano A, et al. Side effects of anabolic androgenic steroids abuse. Int J Sports Med 2008;29(8):679–87.

52. Hartgens F, Rietjens G, Keizer HA, et al. Effects of androgenic-anabolic steroids on apolipoproteins and lipoprotein (a). Br J Sports Med 2004;38(3):253–9.

53. Vogt AM, Geyer H, Jahn L, et al. [Cardiomyopathy associated with uncontrolled self medication of anabolic steroids]. Z Kardiol 2002;91(4):357–62. Kardiomyopathie assoziiert mit unkontrollierter Selbstmedikation anaboler Steroide.

54. Ferenchick GS. Association of steroid abuse with cardiomyopathy in athletes. Am J Med 1991;91(5):562.

55. Payne JR, Kotwinski PJ, Montgomery HE. Cardiac effects of anabolic steroids. Heart 2004;90(5):473–5.

56. Halvorsen S, Thorsby PM, Haug E. [Acute myocardial infarction in a young man who had been using androgenic anabolic steroids]. Tidsskr Nor Laegeforen 2004;124(2):170–2. Akutt hjerteinfarkt hos ung mann som brukte androgene anabole steroider.

57. Fineschi V, Baroldi G, Monciotti F, et al. Anabolic steroid abuse and cardiac sudden death: a pathologic study. Arch Pathol Lab Med 2001;125(2):253–5.

58. Kennedy C. Myocardial infarction in association with misuse of anabolic steroids. Ulster Med J 1993; 62(2):174–6.

59. Lau DH, Stiles MK, John B, et al. Atrial fibrillation and anabolic steroid abuse. Int J Cardiol 2007;117(2):e86–7.

60. Convert O, Duplaa H, Lavielle S, et al. Influence of the replacement of amino acid by its D-enantiomer in the sequence of substance P. 2. Conformational analysis by NMR and energy calculations. Neuropeptides 1991;19(4):259–70.

61. Kanayama G, Hudson JI, Pope HG Jr. Illicit anabolic-androgenic steroid use. Horm Behav 2010;58(1):111–21.

62. Hall RC, Hall RC, Chapman MJ. Psychiatric complications of anabolic steroid abuse. Psychosomatics 2005;46(4):285–90.

63. Talih F, Fattal O, Malone D Jr. Anabolic steroid abuse: psychiatric and physical costs. Cleve Clin J Med 2007;74(5):341–4, 346, 344-349.

64. Pope HG Jr, Katz DL. Affective and psychotic symptoms associated with anabolic steroid use. Am J Psychiatry 1988;145(4):487–90.

65. Parrott AC, Choi PY, Davies M. Anabolic steroid use by amateur athletes: effects upon psychological mood states. J Sports Med Phys Fitness 1994; 34(3):292–8.

66. Cooper CJ, Noakes TD, Dunne T, et al. A high prevalence of abnormal personality traits in chronic users of anabolic-androgenic steroids. Br J Sports Med 1996;30(3):246–50.

67. Kohler TS. Supra-physiologic testosterone supplementation: Do body builders know something we don't?.

68. Pope HG, Kanayama G, Ionescu-Pioggia M, et al. Anabolic steroid users' attitudes towards physicians. Addiction 2004;99(9):1189–94.

69. Selvin E, Feinleib M, Zhang L, et al. Androgens and diabetes in men: results from the Third National Health and Nutrition Examination Survey (NHANES III). Diabetes Care 2007;30(2):234–8.

70. Haffner SM, Shaten J, Stern MP, et al. Low levels of sex hormone-binding globulin and testosterone predict the development of non-insulin-dependent diabetes mellitus in men. MRFIT Research Group. Multiple Risk Factor Intervention Trial. Am J Epidemiol 1996;143(9):889–97.

71. Ding EL, Song Y, Manson JE, et al. Sex hormone-binding globulin and risk of type 2 diabetes in women and men. N Engl J Med 2009;361(12):1152–63.

72. Stellato RK, Feldman HA, Hamdy O, et al. Testosterone, sex hormone-binding globulin, and the development of type 2 diabetes in middle-aged men: prospective results from the Massachusetts male aging study. Diabetes Care 2000;23(4):490–4.

73. Oh JY, Barrett-Connor E, Wedick NM, et al. Endogenous sex hormones and the development of type 2 diabetes in older men and women: the Rancho Bernardo study. Diabetes Care 2002;25(1):55–60.

74. Laaksonen DE, Niskanen L, Punnonen K, et al. Testosterone and sex hormone-binding globulin predict the metabolic syndrome and diabetes in middle-aged men. Diabetes Care 2004;27(5):1036–41.

75. Kelly DM, Jones TH. Testosterone: a vascular hormone in health and disease. J Endocrinol 2013;217(3):R47–71.

76. Hackett G, Cole N, Bhartia M, et al. The response to testosterone undecanoate in men with type 2 diabetes is dependent on achieving threshold serum levels (the BLAST study). Int J Clin Pract 2014;68(2):203–15.

77. Wittert G, Bracken K, Robledo KP, et al. Testosterone treatment to prevent or revert type 2 diabetes in men enrolled in a lifestyle programme (T4DM): a randomised, double-blind, placebo-controlled, 2-year, phase 3b trial. Lancet Diabetes Endocrinol 2021;9(1):32–45.

Benefits and Risks of Testosterone Treatment of Older Men with Hypogonadism

Francesca F. Galbiati, MD[a], Anna L. Goldman, MD[a], Arijeet Gattu, MD[a], Ezgi Caliskan Guzelce, MD[a], Shalender Bhasin, MB, BS[b],*

KEYWORDS

- Aging in men • Men's health • Late-onset hypogonadism • Age-related decline in testosterone
- Benefits of testosterone treatment • Adverse effects of testosterone in older men
- Testosterone replacement in aging men

KEY POINTS

- Circulating total and free testosterone levels decline in men with advancing age.
- In randomized trials, testosterone treatment of older men with low testosterone levels has been associated with improvements in sexual activity, sexual desire, and erectile function; lean body mass, muscle strength, stair climbing power, and self-reported mobility; areal and volumetric bone mineral density, and estimated bone strength; depressive symptoms; and anemia.
- Long-term risks of cardiovascular events and prostate cancer during testosterone treatment remain unclear.

INTRODUCTION

Hypogonadism is a syndrome characterized by a constellation of symptoms and signs associated with the failure of the testis to produce physiologic amounts of testosterone and/or a normal number of spermatozoa due to abnormalities at one or more levels of the hypothalamic-pituitary-testicular (HPT) axis.[1] The term late-onset hypogonadism refers to a cluster of symptoms and signs in older men in association with the age-related decline in testosterone levels similar to those observed in young men with hypogonadism.[1–3] Many cross-sectional and epidemiologic studies agree that total and free testosterone concentrations decline with increasing age in men,[2,4–6] although a few smaller studies of healthy middle-aged and older men who reported excellent or very good health have reported minimal or no change in testosterone levels with advancing age.[7] The trajectory of age-related decline in free testosterone concentrations is greater than that of total testosterone concentrations because sex hormone binding globulin (SHBG) levels increase with advancing age.[4,5,8] The magnitude and rate of age-related decline in total and free testosterone levels is affected by obesity and chronic disease.[9,10] The age-related decline in total and free testosterone levels is associated with sexual symptoms; reduced fat-free mass, muscle strength, self-reported as well as performance-based measures of physical function, mobility limitation, and frailty; depressive symptoms; reduced bone mineral density; and increased risk of diabetes, falls, fractures, and all-cause mortality.[2,11–19] Randomized trials of up to 3 years duration have reported some benefits of testosterone treatment in older men with low testosterone levels and symptoms but long-term safety of testosterone treatment remains to be

[a] Division of Endocrinology, Diabetes, and Hypertension, Brigham and Women's Hospital, 221 Longwood Avenue, Boston, MA 02115, USA; [b] Harvard Medical School, Research Program in Men's Health, Aging and Metabolism, Boston Claude D. Pepper Older Americans Independence Center, Boston, MA, USA
* Corresponding author. Research Program in Men's Health, Aging and Metabolism; Brigham and Women's Hospital, 221 Longwood Avenue, Boston, MA 02115.
E-mail address: SBHASIN@BWH.HARVARD.EDU

Urol Clin N Am 49 (2022) 593–602
https://doi.org/10.1016/j.ucl.2022.07.011
0094-0143/22/© 2022 Elsevier Inc. All rights reserved.

established.[3] Consequently, it has been debated whether older men with age-related decline with testosterone levels should be treated with testosterone. This narrative review presents a critical appraisal of the randomized trials data on the potential benefits and risks of testosterone treatment in older men and offers an individualized, patient-centric approach to a shared treatment decision that is guided by consideration of potential benefits and risks of testosterone treatment, the burden of symptoms, and patient's and clinician's values.

EPIDEMIOLOGY

Men, aged 50 to 65 years, are the most frequent recipients of testosterone prescription,[20] and a sizable proportion of testosterone therapy is being prescribed for age-related decline in testosterone levels, for which testosterone therapy is not approved by the US Food and Drug Administration (FDA).[21] Analyses of data from the Veterans Health Care System[21,22] and Men's Health clinics[23] have revealed that prescription opioid use and anabolic-androgenic steroid use were the most frequent contributors to men receiving a testosterone prescription in the United States. The presence of comorbid conditions, such as obesity, obstructive sleep apnea, depression, and diabetes, and use of antidepressants or systemic glucocorticoids are associated with increased likelihood of receiving a testosterone prescription.[9,21]

Circulating total as well as free testosterone levels in community-dwelling men peak in the second and third decades of life and then decline gradually throughout life (**Fig. 1**).[4,8] Thus, total and free testosterone levels are significantly lower in older men than in young men, but unlike the marked decline in estradiol concentrations during the menopausal transition, there is no discrete inflection point in the age trends for total or free testosterone levels or "andropause" in men. Testosterone concentrations decrease more in men who have greater adiposity, weight gain, and comorbid diseases.[10] Serum luteinizing hormone (LH), follicle stimulating hormone (FSH), and SHBG levels increase with aging.

The proportion of older men whose testosterone levels are below the lower limit of the normal range for healthy young men has varied substantially across epidemiologic studies. Serum testosterone levels in many studies were measured using direct immunoassays that are characterized by high level of imprecision and inaccuracy in the low range. Furthermore, different studies have used varying thresholds of total and/or free testosterone levels to define *hypogonadism* in older men. Also, hypogonadism was defined solely on the basis of low

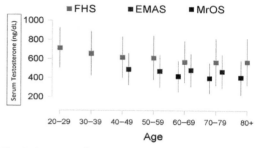

Fig. 1. Mean total testosterone levels expressed in ng/dL (y axis) in the male populations from the Framingham Heart Study (FHS), the European Male Aging Study (EMAS), and the Osteoporotic Fractures in Men (MrOS) study. Serum total testosterone levels measured using liquid chromatography tandem mass spectrometry, in 3 epidemiologic studies: FHS (red), EMAS (blue), and the MrOS study. To convert to SI units (nmol/L), the testosterone concentration in ng/dL should be divided by 28.85. The data are means and 95% confidence intervals. (*From* Travison TG, Vesper HW, Orwoll E, et al. Harmonized reference ranges for circulating testosterone levels in men of four cohort studies in the United States and Europe. J Clin Endocrinol Metab 2017;102(4):1161–173.)

testosterone levels in many studies without consideration of symptoms. Recent studies that have used liquid chromatography tandem mass spectrometry,[2,8,24] the reference method with the highest specificity and accuracy for the measurement of total testosterone levels, have found the prevalence of low testosterone levels to be substantially lower than that reported in older studies, such as the Baltimore Longitudinal Study of Aging.[5] As shown in **Table 1**, only 10% to 14% of men, aged 65 years and older, in the Framingham Heart Study, the Osteoporotic Fractures in Men (MrOS) study, and the European Male Aging Study (EMAS) had serum total testosterone level less than 250 ng/dL (8.7 nmol/L).[2,4,24,25] In the EMAS, the prevalence of late-onset hypogonadism defined by one or more sexual symptoms and a total testosterone level less than 8 nmol/L was 3.2% for men aged 60 to 69 years and 5.1% for those aged 70 to 79 years.[2]

The Healthy Man Study in Australia found no significant age-related decline in testosterone or dihydrotestosterone levels in men who reported being in good or excellent health.[7] The investigators of the Health Man Study have argued that illness, rather than aging itself, is the major contributor to androgen deficiency in older men. However, the subjects enrolled in the Healthy Man Study were not representative of the general population that has high prevalence of obesity and chronic conditions.

Table 1
Percent of community-dwelling older men (age >65 years) with unequivocally low testosterone level from the Framingham Heart Study, the European Male Aging Study, and the Osteoporotic Fracture in Men Study

Study	Number of Men >65 y	Percentage of Men with Total Testosterone Level <250 ng/dL
FHS	1870	12.1
EMAS	1080	7.3
MrOS	2623	10

Age-related decline in testosterone levels are associated with several physiologic changes and age-related conditions[21,23,26–31] (**Box 1**). In epidemiologic studies, total and free serum testosterone levels are positively associated with sexual desire, erectile function, and sexual activity in older men.[2,32] Low total and free testosterone levels are associated with reduced lean body mass, maximal voluntary strength in the upper and lower extremity muscles, and physical function, and increased risk of mobility limitation and frailty.[11–14,16] Age-related decline in testosterone levels is associated with increased risk of anemia. Lowering of testosterone levels by surgical orchiectomy or by administration of a gonadotropin-releasing hormone agonist is associated with progressive loss of bone mineral density and increased fracture risk. Older men with low total and bioavailable testosterone levels are at increased risk of falls, osteoporosis, and fractures.[20–24] Serum estradiol levels are more robustly associated with osteoporosis and fracture risk than total testosterone levels. Low testosterone levels are associated with increased risk of obesity, diabetes mellitus, metabolic syndrome, and dyslipidemia. Testosterone levels are not associated with major depressive syndrome. Middle-aged and older men with low testosterone levels often report depressive symptoms[33]; and low testosterone levels have been associated with late life persistent depressive disorder (dysthymia).[26,27] Testosterone regulates several sexually dimorphic domains of cognition, behaviors, mood, and affect. Although there are inconsistencies among studies, men as a group perform better than women on tests of visuospatial cognition and worse than women on verbal fluency. Preclinical and epidemiologic studies show that testosterone acts as a negative regulator of endogenous Aβ amyloid accumulation in the brain, attenuates tau phosphorylation, reduces neuroinflammation, exerts neuronal protective effect in response to injury and disease, and promotes neuronal regeneration and connectivity.

Box 1
Epidemiologic data on association between testosterone levels and health outcomes and conditions

Health outcomes or conditions with which total or free testosterone levels show a positive association

1. Sexual desire and sexual activity

2. Lean body mass, maximal voluntary strength in the upper and lower extremities, self-reported as well as performance-based measures of physical function

3. Bone mineral density, bone geometry and quality, risk of bone fractures

Health outcomes or conditions with which total or free testosterone levels show a negative association

1. Whole body fat mass and visceral adipose tissue mass

2. Incident diabetes mellitus

3. All-cause mortality and cardiovascular mortality

4. Coronary artery disease, common carotid artery intima-media thickness, high-density lipoprotein cholesterol

5. Risk of falls, frailty, mobility limitation

6. Risk of Alzheimer disease, dementia, fibrillar β-amyloid deposit

7. Late-life low-grade persistent depressive disorder

8. Unexplained anemia in older adults

Health outcomes with which there is weak or inconclusive evidence of association

1. Lower urinary tract symptoms

2. Prostate cancer

3. Major adverse cardiovascular events

4. Major depression

PATHOPHYSIOLOGY OF AGE-RELATED DECLINE IN SERUM TESTOSTERONE LEVELS

Age-related decline in circulating testosterone levels is caused primarily by reduced testosterone production by the testes.[5,18,34–37] Testosterone clearance is lower in older men than in young men.[28] Reduced testosterone production rates in older men are caused by changes affecting all levels of the HPT axis. The diurnal rhythm and pulsatile secretion of testosterone also are altered in older adults, and the synchrony of the frequency and amplitude of pulsatile secretion of LH and testosterone is attenuated in older adults.[7,38–40] HPT axis disturbances are affected by weight gain, chronic illness, medications, and body composition.[9,10] Thus, middle-aged and older adults who experience weight gain, or have chronic diseases, are more likely to have greater decline in testosterone levels than those without weight gain.

POTENTIAL BENEFITS OF TESTOSTERONE TREATMENT IN OLDER MEN: RANDOMIZED CLINICAL TRIALS DATA

Several randomized controlled trials of 3-month to 3-year duration have determined the efficacy of testosterone treatment in older adults. In spite of the heterogeneity of study design, eligibility criteria, the testosterone thresholds, testosterone dose and formulation, end points, and intervention duration, these trials have yielded important information about testosterone's efficacy and safety. Among these trials, the Testosterone Trials (TTrials) was one of the largest, National Institutes of Health-funded, multicenter placebo-controlled trial that was designed to evaluate the efficacy of testosterone treatment in men aged 65 years and older, who had unequivocally low testosterone levels (1 or more of sexual dysfunction, physical dysfunction, or low vitality).[29,30] The TTrials were a coordinated set of 7 placebo-controlled, double-blind trials on 788 men with a mean age of 72 years. Participants had to have an average of 2 fasting, early morning testosterone levels less than 275 ng/dL and low risk for prostate cancer. The eligible participants were allocated by minimization to receive either 1% transdermal testosterone gel or placebo gel for 12 months.[29] Testosterone dose was adjusted based on on-treatment testosterone levels to maintain serum testosterone concentrations between 400 and 700 ng/dL. Testosterone treatment of older men in the Sexual Function Trial of the TTrials was associated with greater improvements in sexual activity across the spectrum from flirting to intercourse, with a moderate effect size of 0.45[29,31] (**Fig. 2**). Testosterone treatment also improved erectile function and sexual desire more than placebo.[31] Meta-analyses of placebo-controlled trials have reported significantly greater improvements in sexual activity, sexual desire, erectile function, and satisfaction with sexual experience with testosterone treatment than with placebo.[34] Testosterone treatment does not, however, improve sexual function in asymptomatic men or in men who do not have low testosterone levels.[35] Testosterone treatment has not been shown to improve ejaculatory function in men with ejaculatory dysfunction.[36] Testosterone's effects on erectile response to phosphodiesterase-5 (PDE5)

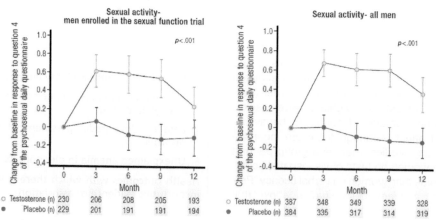

Fig. 2. Effect of testosterone on sexual activity in the participants of the TTrials. Change from baseline in sexual activity in (*left*) men taking testosterone or placebo and enrolled in the Sexual Function Trial and (*right*) all men enrolled in the TTrials. Data are presented as means and 95% confidence intervals. (*From* Snyder PJ, Bhasin S, Cunningham GR, et al. Testosterone Trials I. Effects of testosterone treatment in older men. N Engl J Med 2016;374(7):611–24.)

inhibitors remain incompletely understood[37]; the improvement in erectile function in response to PDE5 inhibitors, such as sildenafil, alone is substantial and further addition of testosterone has not been shown to further improve erectile function relative to placebo[37] (**Table 2**).

Testosterone treatment increases lean body mass, maximal voluntary muscle strength, and muscle power in healthy young men, hypogonadal men, healthy older men, and older men with functional limitations and chronic diseases such as that associated with chronic obstructive lung disease and human immunodeficiency virus-associated weight loss.[38,41–50] Testosterone's effects on lean body mass and maximal voluntary muscle strength are related to the administered dose and circulating testosterone concentrations in young as well as older men.[39,40] Testosterone's effects on muscle performance are domain specific; testosterone increases muscle strength and power, but it does not improve muscle fatigability or specific force.[44] Testosterone treatment improves self-reported physical function,[51] but its effects on performance-based measures of physical function have been inconsistent across trials.[38,44,48,49,52,53] The performance-based measures of physical function that are more robustly related to lower-extremity muscle strength and power such as the stair climbing speed and power have shown consistent improvements with testosterone treatment in randomized trial.[38] However, testosterone's effects on walking speed have been small and inconsistent across trials.

The Physical Function Trial (PFT) of the TTrials determined the effects of testosterone treatment on mobility and self-reported physical function in older men with low testosterone concentrations, self-reported mobility limitation, and walking speed less than 1.2 m/s. The 6-minute walking distance improved significantly more in the testosterone than in the placebo group among all men in the TTrials, but not in those who were enrolled in the PFT. Testosterone treatment was associated with greater improvements in the self-reported physical function, assessed using the physical component of the Medical Outcomes Study Short Form-36 (PF10), than the placebo treatment in all men in TTrials and in men enrolled in the PFT. A greater proportion of men in the testosterone group reported that their walking ability had improved than men in the placebo group. The changes in 6-minute walking distance in testosterone-treated men were related to changes in testosterone level as well as the hemoglobin level.

In the Bone Trial of the TTrials, testosterone treatment was associated with greater improvements in vertebral and femoral volumetric as well as areal bone mineral density and estimated bone strength than placebo. The improvements in volumetric bone mineral density were greater in the spine than hip and more in the trabecular than peripheral bone.[54] Meta-analyses of randomized trials also have reported significant improvements in vertebral bone mineral density with testosterone treatment, with greater improvements in bone mineral density in trials that used intramuscular rather than transdermal testosterone gels.[55] None of the trials, however, has been sufficient large or long to evaluate the effects of testosterone treatment on bone fractures.[53]

Testosterone increases hemoglobin and red blood cell counts. In the TTrials as well as in the Testosterone in Older Men (TOM Trial) Trial, testosterone treatment of older men with unexplained anemia of aging was associated with a higher proportion of participants correcting their anemia during the intervention period than that associated with placebo.[56,57] In the TTrials, testosterone-induced increase in hemoglobin levels was associated with improvements in 6-minute walking distance and vitality.[56]

Testosterone treatment has a modest effect in improving depressive symptoms in middle-aged and older men with testosterone deficiency.[58,59] However, testosterone treatment is not efficacious in treating major depressive disorder. Small randomized trials in middle-aged and older men with late-onset persistent depressive disorder (dysthymia) have reported greater improvements with testosterone treatment compared with placebo in depressive symptoms.[60,61] Randomized trials have not shown a clear benefit of

Table 2 Effects of testosterone replacement therapy on different systems from the TTrials	
Impact	**No Impact**
Bone mineral density	Vitality
Sexual feelings and thoughts	Distance walked in 6 min
Sexual activity	Cognitive function
Number of spontaneous erections	
Anemia of known and unknown cause	
Depressive symptoms	
Self-reported walking distance	
Gait speed	

testosterone treatment in alleviating fatigue in older adults.[29,30,49] However, one large trial of a testosterone solution reported significantly greater improvements in energy in hypogonadal men with low energy.[62]

Testosterone's effects on insulin sensitivity and glycemic control have varied across studies. In the T4DM Trial,[63] a randomized, placebo-controlled trial, men, aged 50 to 74 years, a serum testosterone concentration of 402 ng/dL (14.0 nmol/L) or lower, and impaired glucose tolerance (oral glucose tolerance test 2-hour glucose 141–200 mg/dL) or newly diagnosed type 2 diabetes were enrolled in a lifestyle program and randomly assigned to receive an intramuscular injection of testosterone undecanoate (1000 mg) or placebo for 2 years. Testosterone treatment for 2 years was associated with a lower proportion of participants with type 2 diabetes compared with the lifestyle program alone. The participants in the T4DM trial were not hypogonadal.

POTENTIAL RISKS OF TESTOSTERONE TREATMENT

Older men may be at increased risk of testosterone's adverse effects than young men for several reasons. The apparent metabolic clearance of testosterone is lower in older men than in young men resulting in higher circulating testosterone level, after adjusting for the administered dose.[28] Older men exhibit greater increases in hemoglobin and hematocrit than young men even after adjusting for the administered dose and testosterone levels.[64] Testosterone treatment of carefully selected older men in randomized trials has been associated with a low frequency of adverse events and serious adverse events.[34] Erythrocytosis is the most common adverse effect reported in randomized trials of testosterone.[34] Other adverse effects include acne, oiliness of skin, breast tenderness, leg edema, suppression of spermatogenesis, and infertility.[1] Testosterone treatment does not worsen lower urinary tract symptoms in middle-aged and older men who do not have severe lower urinary tract symptoms at baseline.[65] Also, randomized trials have not provided clear evidence of the association of testosterone treatment with the development of gynecomastia or the worsening of obstructive sleep apnea.

Concerns about the potential risk of an increase in cardiovascular events and prostate cancer with testosterone treatment have been a source of much controversy. None of the trials has been of sufficient size or duration to have adequate statistical power for determining the effects of testosterone treatment on major adverse cardiovascular events or prostate cancer events. Hypogonadal men have lower prostate specific antigen (PSA) levels than eugonadal men, and testosterone treatment of older men with hypogonadism increases serum PSA levels by an average of .44 ng/mL.[66] PSA levels fluctuate over time due to biological factors as well as assay variation; PSA elevations in some men will lead to prostate biopsy. Because of the high prevalence of subclinical prostate cancer in older men, a prostate biopsy increases the likelihood of detection of a subclinical prostate cancer. Thus, older men receiving testosterone treatment are at increased risk of being referred for a prostate biopsy and of the detection of a subclinical prostate cancer.[66]

Testosterone treatment exerts many diverse physiologic effects on cardiovascular system in men; some of these effects could potentially increase the risk of cardiovascular events, whereas others could reduce the risk of such events. Testosterone increases hemoglobin and hematocrit, causes salt and water retention that can worsen preexisting heart failure, and induces platelet aggregation, all of which could potentially increase cardiovascular risk. Testosterone also is a potent vasodilator and increases coronary blood flow; reduces whole body and visceral adiposity, and improves insulin sensitivity in some experimental models. In the Testosterone's Effects on Atherosclerosis Progression in Aging Men (The TEAAM Trial), testosterone treatment of middle-aged and older men for 3 years had no significant effect on atherosclerosis progression, assessed by measuring common carotid artery intima media thickness and coronary calcium scores using the multidetector computed tomography.[35] In the Cardiovascular Trial of the TTrials,[67] testosterone treatment for 1 year was associated with a greater increase in the volume of noncalcified soft coronary artery plaque measured using computed tomographic angiography compared with placebo, but the change in coronary artery calcium score did not differ between the testosterone and placebo groups. An individual patient-level meta-analysis of randomized trials did not find a significant difference in the incidence of cardiovascular events between testosterone or placebo arms.[68] The retrospective analyses of pharmacovigilance studies and electronic medical records have been inconclusive because of the inherent limitations of such studies, including the heterogeneity of study populations, eligibility criteria, variable testosterone doses and intervention durations, and end points. Importantly, none of the randomized trials, with the exception of the TTrials, prospectively ascertained major adverse cardiovascular events using a standardized adjudication protocol. The number of adjudicated MACE in the TTrials was too small to permit meaningful evaluation. Careful analyses of the available data by the FDA and European Medicine Agency concluded that there was insufficient evidence of increased cardiovascular risk in testosterone trials. However, the FDA required that the manufacturers of testosterone products add information to the drug label about a possible increased risk of heart attacks and strokes.

Fortunately, a large randomized, placebo-controlled trial is currently underway to determine the effects of testosterone replacement therapy on the incidence of adjudicated major adverse cardiovascular events in men, aged 45 to 80 years, who meet the Endocrine Society criteria for hypogonadism (The TRAVERSE Trial NCT NCT03518034).[69] Because of its large sample size (up to 6000 men) and long intervention duration (up to 5 years), the trial also will provide important information about the risk of high-grade prostate cancer and the efficacy of testosterone treatment in improving progression from prediabetes to diabetes, depressive symptoms, correcting anemia of aging, sexual symptoms, and clinical fractures.[69]

A PATIENT-CENTRIC APPROACH BASED ON CONSIDERATION OF INDIVIDUALIZED BENEFITS AND RISKS AND VALUES

Total and free testosterone levels in men decline with aging; 3% to 5% of middle-aged and older men have low testosterone levels and one or more sexual symptoms. Randomized trials of 1 to 3 years duration have provided evidence of some benefits, although the long-term safety of testosterone with respect to the risk of cardiovascular events and prostate cancer remains unknown. In randomized trials, testosterone treatment of older men with low testosterone levels and one or more symptoms have reported improvements in sexual symptoms; volumetric and areal bone mineral density and estimated bone strength; lean body mass, muscle strength, and stair climbing power; and depressive symptoms. Testosterone treatment is also efficacious in correcting unexplained anemia in older adults. Testosterone's effects on hard clinically important outcomes such as fractures, falls, progression from prediabetes to diabetes, late-onset persistent low-grade depressive disorder, and physical disability remain unknown.

In light of the uncertainty about long-term safety of testosterone treatment, an expert panel of the Endocrine Society did not recommend testosterone treatment of *all* older men with low testosterone levels. Instead, the panel suggested that "...in older men, who have symptoms or conditions suggestive of testosterone deficiency (such as low libido or unexplained anemia) and consistently and unequivocally low morning testosterone concentrations, clinicians offer testosterone therapy on an individualized basis after explicit discussion of the potential risks and benefits." The decision to treat older men with testosterone should be guided by consideration of additional complexities. The burden of symptoms should be weighed against the uncertainties of long-term adverse effects. The level of imprecision and inaccuracy should be considered in the diagnosis of hypogonadism especially when testosterone levels are within 2 SDs of the diagnostic thresholds of testosterone levels. One should evaluate whether the patient has conditions such as history of prostate cancer, breast cancer, heart failure, venous thromboembolic event, recent MACE) that might increase the risk of harm. It should be recognized that screening and monitoring for prostate cancer in men with hypogonadism receiving testosterone treatment has the potential of causing harm. Therefore, the decision to offer testosterone replacement therapy to older men should be a shared decision based on an individualized assessment of potential benefits and risks and consideration of the patient's as well as the clinician's values.

CLINICS CARE POINTS

- The diagnosis of testosterone deficiency should be made only in men with consistently low total and/or free testosterone levels, measured using reliable assays, and associated signs and symptoms. One should evaluate for the presence of conditions that might increase the potential for harm during testosterone treatment.

- The decision to treat should be guided by consideration of the burden of symptoms, individualized assessment of potential benefits and risks, and patient's and clinician's values.

- Testosterone treatment should be associated with a standardized monitoring plan. Screening and monitoring for prostate cancer has the potential for harm. Therefore, decision to treat and monitor for prostate cancer should be a shared decision.

DISCLOSURE

Dr S. Bhasin reports receiving research grants from NIA, NINR, NICHD/NCMRR, AbbVie, MIB, FPT, and Transition Therapeutics, and consulting fees from Aditum and OPKO. These conflicts are managed according to regulations of the Office of Industry Interaction, MGB Healthcare System.

REFERENCES

1. Bhasin S, Brito JP, Cunningham GR, et al. Testosterone Therapy in Men With Hypogonadism: An Endocrine Society Clinical Practice Guideline. J Clin Endocrinol Metab 2018;103(5):1715–44.
2. Wu FC, Tajar A, Beynon JM, et al. Identification of late-onset hypogonadism in middle-aged and elderly men. N Engl J Med 2010;363(2):123–35.
3. Bhasin S. Testosterone replacement in aging men: an evidence-based patient-centric perspective. J Clin Invest 2021;131(4):e146607.
4. Bhasin S, Pencina M, Jasuja GK, et al. Reference ranges for testosterone in men generated using liquid chromatography tandem mass spectrometry in a community-based sample of healthy nonobese young men in the Framingham Heart Study and applied to three geographically distinct cohorts. J Clin Endocrinol Metab 2011;96(8):2430–9.
5. Harman SM, Metter EJ, Tobin JD, et al. Baltimore Longitudinal Study of A. Longitudinal effects of aging on serum total and free testosterone levels in healthy men. Baltimore Longitudinal Study of Aging. J Clin Endocrinol Metab 2001;86(2):724–31.
6. Travison TG, Araujo AB, Kupelian V, et al. The relative contributions of aging, health, and lifestyle factors to serum testosterone decline in men. J Clin Endocrinol Metab 2007;92(2):549–55.
7. Sartorius G, Spasevska S, Idan A, et al. Serum testosterone, dihydrotestosterone and estradiol concentrations in older men self-reporting very good health: the healthy man study. Clin Endocrinol (Oxf) 2012;77(5):755–63.
8. Travison TG, Vesper HW, Orwoll E, et al. Harmonized Reference Ranges for Circulating Testosterone Levels in Men of Four Cohort Studies in the United States and Europe. J Clin Endocrinol Metab 2017; 102(4):1161–73.
9. Tajar A, Forti G, O'Neill TW, et al. Characteristics of secondary, primary, and compensated hypogonadism in aging men: evidence from the European Male Ageing Study. J Clin Endocrinol Metab 2010; 95(4):1810–8.
10. Mohr BA, Bhasin S, Link CL, et al. The effect of changes in adiposity on testosterone levels in older men: longitudinal results from the Massachusetts Male Aging Study. Eur J Endocrinol 2006;155(3): 443–52.
11. Roy TA, Blackman MR, Harman SM, et al. Interrelationships of serum testosterone and free testosterone index with FFM and strength in aging men. Am J Physiol Endocrinol Metab 2002;283(2): E284–94.
12. Baumgartner RN, Waters DL, Gallagher D, et al. Predictors of skeletal muscle mass in elderly men and women. Mech Ageing Dev 1999;107(2): 123–36.
13. Krasnoff JB, Basaria S, Pencina MJ, et al. Free testosterone levels are associated with mobility limitation and physical performance in community-dwelling men: the Framingham Offspring Study. J Clin Endocrinol Metab 2010;95(6):2790–9.
14. Schaap LA, Pluijm SM, Deeg DJ, et al. Low testosterone levels and decline in physical performance and muscle strength in older men: findings from two prospective cohort studies. Clin Endocrinol (Oxf) 2008;68(1):42–50.
15. Araujo AB, Dixon JM, Suarez EA, et al. Clinical review: Endogenous testosterone and mortality in men: a systematic review and meta-analysis. J Clin Endocrinol Metab 2011;96(10):3007–19.
16. Vandenput L, Mellstrom D, Laughlin GA, et al. Low Testosterone, but Not Estradiol, Is Associated With Incident Falls in Older Men: The International MrOS Study. J Bone Miner Res 2017;32(6):1174–81.
17. Ding EL, Song Y, Malik VS, et al. Sex differences of endogenous sex hormones and risk of type 2 diabetes: a systematic review and meta-analysis. JAMA 2006;295(11):1288–99.
18. Hsu B, Cumming RG, Seibel MJ, et al. Reproductive Hormones and Longitudinal Change in Bone Mineral Density and Incident Fracture Risk in Older Men: The Concord Health and Aging in Men Project. J Bone Miner Res 2015;30(9):1701–8.
19. Cawthon PM, Schousboe JT, Harrison SL, et al. Osteoporotic Fractures in Men Study Research G. Sex hormones, sex hormone binding globulin, and vertebral fractures in older men. Bone 2016;84: 271–8.
20. Nguyen CP, Hirsch MS, Moeny D, et al. Testosterone and "Age-Related Hypogonadism"–FDA Concerns. N Engl J Med 2015;373(8):689–91.
21. Jasuja GK, Bhasin S, Reisman JI, et al. Who Gets Testosterone? Patient Characteristics Associated with Testosterone Prescribing in the Veteran Affairs System: a Cross-Sectional Study. J Gen Intern Med 2017;32(3):304–11.
22. Jasuja GK, Ameli O, Reisman JI, et al. Health Outcomes Among Long-term Opioid Users With Testosterone Prescription in the Veterans Health Administration. JAMA Netw Open 2019;2(12): e1917141.
23. Coward RM, Rajanahally S, Kovac JR, et al. Anabolic steroid induced hypogonadism in young men. J Urol 2013;190(6):2200–5.

24. Orwoll E, Lambert LC, Marshall LM, et al. Testosterone and estradiol among older men. J Clin Endocrinol Metab 2006;91(4):1336–44.

25. Liverman CT, Blazer DG, editors. eds Testosterone and Aging: Clinical Research Directions. Washington, DC: National Academies Press; 2004.

26. Seidman SN, Araujo AB, Roose SP, et al. Low testosterone levels in elderly men with dysthymic disorder. Am J Psychiatry 2002;159(3):456–9.

27. Shores MM, Sloan KL, Matsumoto AM, et al. Increased incidence of diagnosed depressive illness in hypogonadal older men. Arch Gen Psychiatry 2004;61(2):162–7.

28. Coviello AD, Lakshman K, Mazer NA, et al. Differences in the apparent metabolic clearance rate of testosterone in young and older men with gonadotropin suppression receiving graded doses of testosterone. J Clin Endocrinol Metab 2006;91(11):4669–75.

29. Snyder PJ, Bhasin S, Cunningham GR, et al. Testosterone Trials I. Effects of Testosterone Treatment in Older Men. N Engl J Med 2016;374(7):611–24.

30. Snyder PJ, Bhasin S, Cunningham GR, et al. Lessons From the Testosterone Trials. Endocr Rev 2018;39(3):369–86.

31. Cunningham GR, Stephens-Shields AJ, Rosen RC, et al. Testosterone Treatment and Sexual Function in Older Men With Low Testosterone Levels. J Clin Endocrinol Metab 2016;101(8):3096–104.

32. Cunningham GR, Stephens-Shields AJ, Rosen RC, et al. Association of sex hormones with sexual function, vitality, and physical function of symptomatic older men with low testosterone levels at baseline in the testosterone trials. J Clin Endocrinol Metab 2015;100(3):1146–55.

33. Khera M, Bhattacharya RK, Blick G, et al. The effect of testosterone supplementation on depression symptoms in hypogonadal men from the Testim Registry in the US (TRiUS). Aging Male 2012;15(1):14–21.

34. Ponce OJ, Spencer-Bonilla G, Alvarez-Villalobos N, et al. The efficacy and adverse events of testosterone replacement therapy in hypogonadal men: A systematic review and meta-analysis of randomized, placebo-controlled trials. J Clin Endocrinol Metab 2018. https://doi.org/10.1210/jc.2018-00404.

35. Basaria S, Harman SM, Travison TG, et al. Effects of Testosterone Administration for 3 Years on Subclinical Atherosclerosis Progression in Older Men With Low or Low-Normal Testosterone Levels: A Randomized Clinical Trial. JAMA 2015;314(6):570–81.

36. Paduch DA, Polzer PK, Ni X, et al. Testosterone Replacement in Androgen-Deficient Men With Ejaculatory Dysfunction: A Randomized Controlled Trial. J Clin Endocrinol Metab 2015;100(8):2956–62.

37. Spitzer M, Basaria S, Travison TG, et al. Effect of testosterone replacement on response to sildenafil citrate in men with erectile dysfunction: a parallel, randomized trial. Ann Intern Med 2012;157(10):681–91.

38. Storer TW, Basaria S, Traustadottir T, et al. Effects of Testosterone Supplementation for 3 Years on Muscle Performance and Physical Function in Older Men. J Clin Endocrinol Metab 2017;102(2):583–93.

39. Bhasin S, Woodhouse L, Casaburi R, et al. Testosterone dose-response relationships in healthy young men. Am J Physiol Endocrinol Metab 2001;281(6):E1172–81.

40. Bhasin S, Woodhouse L, Casaburi R, et al. Older men are as responsive as young men to the anabolic effects of graded doses of testosterone on the skeletal muscle. J Clin Endocrinol Metab 2005;90(2):678–88.

41. Bhasin S, Storer TW, Berman N, et al. The effects of supraphysiologic doses of testosterone on muscle size and strength in normal men. N Engl J Med 1996;335(1):1–7.

42. Bhasin S, Storer TW, Berman N, et al. Testosterone replacement increases fat-free mass and muscle size in hypogonadal men. J Clin Endocrinol Metab 1997;82(2):407–13.

43. Bhasin S, Storer TW, Javanbakht M, et al. Testosterone replacement and resistance exercise in HIV-infected men with weight loss and low testosterone levels. JAMA 2000;283(6):763–70.

44. Storer TW, Magliano L, Woodhouse L, et al. Testosterone dose-dependently increases maximal voluntary strength and leg power, but does not affect fatigability or specific tension. J Clin Endocrinol Metab 2003;88(4):1478–85.

45. Casaburi R, Bhasin S, Cosentino L, et al. Effects of testosterone and resistance training in men with chronic obstructive pulmonary disease. Am J Respir Crit Care Med 2004;170(8):870–8.

46. Grinspoon S, Corcoran C, Askari H, et al. Effects of androgen administration in men with the AIDS wasting syndrome. A randomized, double-blind, placebo-controlled trial. Ann Intern Med 1998;129(1):18–26.

47. Knapp PE, Storer TW, Herbst KL, et al. Effects of a supraphysiological dose of testosterone on physical function, muscle performance, mood, and fatigue in men with HIV-associated weight loss. Am J Physiol Endocrinol Metab 2008;294(6):E1135–43.

48. Srinivas-Shankar U, Roberts SA, Connolly MJ, et al. Effects of testosterone on muscle strength, physical function, body composition, and quality of life in intermediate-frail and frail elderly men: a randomized, double-blind, placebo-controlled study. J Clin Endocrinol Metab 2010;95(2):639–50.

49. Travison TG, Basaria S, Storer TW, et al. Clinical meaningfulness of the changes in muscle performance and physical function associated with testosterone administration in older men with mobility

limitation. J Gerontol A Biol Sci Med Sci 2011;66(10): 1090–9.

50. Traustadottir T, Harman SM, Tsitouras P, et al. Long-Term Testosterone Supplementation in Older Men Attenuates Age-Related Decline in Aerobic Capacity. J Clin Endocrinol Metab 2018;103(8):2861–9.

51. Bhasin S, Ellenberg SS, Storer TW, et al. Effect of testosterone replacement on measures of mobility in older men with mobility limitation and low testosterone concentrations: secondary analyses of the Testosterone Trials. Lancet Diabetes Endocrinol 2018;6(11):879–90.

52. Nair KS, Rizza RA, O'Brien P, et al. DHEA in elderly women and DHEA or testosterone in elderly men. N Engl J Med 2006;355(16):1647–59.

53. Emmelot-Vonk MH, Verhaar HJ, Nakhai Pour HR, et al. Effect of testosterone supplementation on functional mobility, cognition, and other parameters in older men: a randomized controlled trial. JAMA 2008;299(1):39–52.

54. Snyder PJ, Kopperdahl DL, Stephens-Shields AJ, et al. Effect of Testosterone Treatment on Volumetric Bone Density and Strength in Older Men With Low Testosterone: A Controlled Clinical Trial. JAMA Intern Med 2017;177(4):471–9.

55. Tracz MJ, Sideras K, Bolona ER, et al. Testosterone use in men and its effects on bone health. A systematic review and meta-analysis of randomized placebo-controlled trials. J Clin Endocrinol Metab 2006;91(6):2011–6.

56. Roy CN, Snyder PJ, Stephens-Shields AJ, et al. Association of Testosterone Levels With Anemia in Older Men: A Controlled Clinical Trial. JAMA Intern Med 2017;177(4):480–90.

57. Bachman E, Travison TG, Basaria S, et al. Testosterone induces erythrocytosis via increased erythropoietin and suppressed hepcidin: evidence for a new erythropoietin/hemoglobin set point. J Gerontol A Biol Sci Med Sci 2014;69(6):725–35.

58. Walther A, Breidenstein J, Miller R. Association of Testosterone Treatment With Alleviation of Depressive Symptoms in Men: A Systematic Review and Meta-analysis. JAMA Psychiatry 2019;76(1):31–40.

59. Bhasin S, Seidman S. Testosterone Treatment of Depressive Disorders in Men: Too Much Smoke, Not Enough High-Quality Evidence. JAMA Psychiatry 2019;76(1):9–10.

60. Seidman SN, Orr G, Raviv G, et al. Effects of testosterone replacement in middle-aged men with dysthymia: a randomized, placebo-controlled clinical trial. J Clin Psychopharmacol 2009;29(3):216–21.

61. Shores MM, Kivlahan DR, Sadak TI, et al. A randomized, double-blind, placebo-controlled study of testosterone treatment in hypogonadal older men with subthreshold depression (dysthymia or minor depression). J Clin Psychiatry 2009;70(7): 1009–16.

62. Brock G, Heiselman D, Maggi M, et al. Effect of Testosterone Solution 2% on Testosterone Concentration, Sex Drive and Energy in Hypogonadal Men: Results of a Placebo Controlled Study. J Urol 2016;195(3):699–705.

63. Wittert G, Bracken K, Robledo KP, et al. Testosterone treatment to prevent or revert type 2 diabetes in men enrolled in a lifestyle programme (T4DM): a randomised, double-blind, placebo-controlled, 2-year, phase 3b trial. Lancet Diabetes Endocrinol 2021; 9(1):32–45.

64. Coviello AD, Kaplan B, Lakshman KM, et al. Effects of graded doses of testosterone on erythropoiesis in healthy young and older men. J Clin Endocrinol Metab 2008;93(3):914–9.

65. Kathrins M, Doersch K, Nimeh T, et al. The Relationship Between Testosterone-Replacement Therapy and Lower Urinary Tract Symptoms: A Systematic Review. Urology 2016;88:22–32.

66. Calof OM, Singh AB, Lee ML, et al. Adverse events associated with testosterone replacement in middle-aged and older men: a meta-analysis of randomized, placebo-controlled trials. J Gerontol A Biol Sci Med Sci 2005;60(11):1451–7.

67. Budoff MJ, Ellenberg SS, Lewis CE, et al. Testosterone Treatment and Coronary Artery Plaque Volume in Older Men With Low Testosterone. JAMA 2017;317(7):708–16.

68. Hudson J, Cruickshank M, Quinton R, et al. Adverse cardiovascular events and mortality in men during testosterone treatment: an individual patient and aggregate data meta-analysis. Lancet Healthy Longev 2022;3(6):e381–93.

69. Bhasin S, Lincoff AM, Basaria S, et al. Effects of long-term testosterone treatment on cardiovascular outcomes in men with hypogonadism: Rationale and design of the TRAVERSE study. Am Heart J 2022;245:41–50.

Testosterone and the Androgen Receptor

Thomas Gerald, MD*, Ganesh Raj, MD, PhD

KEYWORDS

- Testosterone ● Androgen receptor ● Dihydrotestosterone ● Structure ● Function

KEY POINTS

- Testosterone is a critical steroid hormone involved in the development of male sexual characteristics and function as well as regulation of many homeostatic mechanisms throughout life.
- The production and metabolism of testosterone is tightly regulated by the hypothalamic-pituitary (HPG) axis in order to maintain strict homeostasis among the involved physiologic processes.
- Additional steroid hormones involved in testosterone steroidogenesis and metabolism, including dihydrotestosterone and estradiol, occupy an important position in exerting effects on target tissues and in regulating the HPG axis.
- When activated by androgens, the androgen receptor is involved in genomic and nongenomic signal transduction to exert the intended effect on the target tissue.

INTRODUCTION

The steroid hormone testosterone is among the most widely studied in the endocrine system. Testosterone is the major sex hormone in men and critically influences male development and maintenance of physiologic functions of multiple organ systems across all ages, including in sexual differentiation, development of male secondary sexual organs, sperm production, libido, muscle size and strength, and bone growth and strength. The male phenotype strongly depends on the expression of testosterone and its byproducts. Adolescent boys with too little testosterone may not experience normal masculinization. In contrast, athletes who use anabolic steroids, testosterone, or related hormones to increase muscle mass and athletic performance have abnormally high testosterone levels.

Testosterone levels are carefully regulated by an elegant multitier feedback system with positive and negative feedback mechanisms that tightly regulate hormonal levels and expected physiologic changes. Testosterone is the ligand for the androgen receptor (AR), which produces its effects through regulation of both gene transcription and translation of proteins as well as through second messenger systems for both prolonged and rapid effects.

HISTORICAL EFFECTS OF TESTOSTERONE

The biological effects of the testes and testosterone have been known since antiquity. In Greek mythology, the titan Chronos castrates his father Uranos. Aristotle knew the effects of castration on reproductive biology. Castration has been performed as punishment and to produce obedient slaves but also to preserve the soprano voices of prepubertal boys. Imperial courts used castrated men as overseers in harems. In multiple cultures, testicles from various animals were consumed to

Funding: This article was made possible by funding to GVR from the Simmons Cancer Center at UT Southwestern for the Prostate Cancer Program, the Mimi and John Cole Prostate Cancer Fund, the Wilson Foundation and the Department of Defense Grants W81XWH-17-1-0674, W81XWH-19-1-0363, and W81XWH-21-1-0687.
Department of Urology, University of Texas Southwestern Medical Center, 5323 Harry Hines Boulevard, Dallas, TX 75390-9110, USA
* Corresponding author.
E-mail address: Thomas.Gerald@UTSouthwestern.edu

improve virility.[1] In 1786, John Hunter transplanted testes into capons in London, without understanding the implications of the endocrine aspects. Arnold Berthold in Gottingen, Germany in 1849 observed that castrated roosters failed to develop expected secondary sexual characteristics, including development of the comb, aggressive behavior, crowing, muscle development, and sexual interest in hens. Berthold then showed that transplantation of testes back into two roosters resulted in remasculinization and appearance of secondary sexual characteristics.[2,3] From these systematic studies, Berthold established the role of internal secretion from the testicular transplantations as regulators of sexual characteristics and is considered as the father of modern endocrinology.

In 1889, Charles E. Brown-Séquard famously reported on 10 subcutaneous self-injections of the combination of testicular vein blood, semen, and testicular extract from dogs and guinea pigs. He reported an astonishing self-described recovery of endurance, strength, cognition, and even urinary and bowel function.[4] An analysis finding that the small amount of testosterone extracted by this method has pointed authors to conclude that Brown-Sequard likely experienced a placebo effect.[5] However, the explosion of interest in the Western world in the use of animal organ extracts that subsequently occurred resulted in the springing up of factories in Europe and America for its production and thousands of physicians engaging in their prescription. This perfectly illustrates the fascination in the medical community and popular culture alike with restoration of male function and virility.[2,3,5] Indeed, the twentieth century witnessed a steady progression in the understanding of male androgen function with the crystalline isolation of testosterone by Ernst Laqueur from bovine testes in 1935. Laquer was the first to call the male androgenic hormone "testosterone." In the same year testosterone was chemically synthesized independently by Adolf Butenandt in Göttingen and Leopold Ruzicka in Basel, a feat that was recognized by their joint Nobel prize in chemistry in 1939. The development of synthetic, longer acting, injectable testosterone enanthate preparations in the 1950s enabled widespread usage of synthetic testosterone.[1-3] Currently, there continues to be increasing interest and the use of testosterone replacement among men of all age groups, with more than 4-fold increases in the number of men using testosterone replacement during the first decade of this century.[6,7]

ANDROGEN STEROIDOGENESIS FROM CHOLESTEROL

The primary site of testosterone production is the Leydig cell within the testis, resulting in 95% of circulating testosterone being produced by the testes.[8] Cholesterol is used as a precursor and is produced de novo within the cell or acquired via lipoprotein receptors. Cholesterol can either then be stored as an ester or transferred to the mitochondrial membrane by steroidogenic acute regulatory protein for steroid synthesis. A series of synthetic steps occurs ultimately resulting in testosterone (**Fig. 1**).[8,9] Leydig cells preferentially express a specific isoform of 17β-hydroxysteroid dehydrogenase (HSD), which favors the conversion of androstenedione to testosterone.[10] Additionally, Leydig cells produce small amounts of other steroid hormones in this pathway including dihydrotestosterone (DHT), dehydroepiandrosterone, androstenedione, estradiol, estrone, and progesterone.[11]

TESTOSTERONE REGULATION, PRODUCTION, AND TRANSPORT

Testosterone is under the regulation of the hypothalamic-pituitary-gonadal (HPG) axis (**Fig. 2**). In this classic positive and negative feedback system, gonadotropin-releasing hormone (GnRH) is released into the hypophyseal portal system by hypothalamic neurons responding kisspeptin stimulation from neighboring neurons.[12,13] GnRH stimulates production and release of luteinizing hormone (LH) and follicle-stimulating hormone from the anterior pituitary. Leydig cells express the LH receptor, and through this, LH exerts a steroidogenic effect for testosterone production and trophic effect promoting Leydig cell growth and proliferation. Testosterone and estradiol then provide negative feedback at the level of the hypothalamus and pituitary to limit GnRH and LH production.[14,15]

Testosterone produced within the Leydig cell has 2 ultimate fates: remain within the seminiferous tubule to optimize spermatogenesis or enter circulation to exert its effect on distant tissues.[8,9,16] Local diffusion within the seminiferous tubule is mediated by androgen-binding protein, resulting in a significantly higher testosterone levels within the luminal compartment when compared with circulating levels.[17] These levels optimize spermatogenesis by Sertoli cells and sperm function through independent and estradiol-mediated mechanisms. Within the peripheral circulation, testosterone reaches equilibrium with the serum proteins: 60% bound tightly

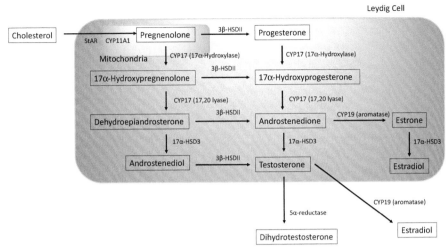

Fig. 1. Androgen steroidogenesis. Cholesterol is the precursor for androgen synthesis and is transported into the cell by lipoprotein receptors. It is transported to the mitochondrial membrane by steroidogenic acute regulatory protein. CYP17, 3β-HSDII, and 17α-HSD3 are involved with subsequent synthesis steps for testosterone. Testosterone may then enter the circulation and act primarily on target tissues or be converted to DHT or estradiol peripherally by 5AR and aromatase, respectively.

bound to sex hormone binding globulin (SHBG), 38% weakly bound to albumin, and 2% unbound. The proportion of testosterone that is bound to albumin and free is considered the bioavailable component.[18] SHBG is produced in the liver, and its circulating levels can be influenced by medications and disease states. Estrogen, tamoxifen, antiepileptic drugs, age, and hyperthyroidism can increase SHBG levels, although exogenous androgen, glucocorticoid, or growth hormone therapy, untreated hypothyroidism, obesity, and hyperinsulinemic states may decrease SHBG. Alterations in SHBG levels in turn cause corresponding effects in the bioavailability of testosterone to target tissues, and polymorphisms and expression levels of SHBG may be associated with reduced fertility, erectile dysfunction, and late-onset hypogonadism as well as prostate cancer incidence and prognosis.[19,20]

TESTOSTERONE VARIATION AND FUNCTION

Androgens drive a variety of biologic effects throughout an individual's lifetime. There are 3 peaks of testosterone activity: during fetal life, as a neonate, and during puberty (**Fig. 3**).[16] During the fetal peak, testosterone production is under the control of maternal hCG and fetal LH. Testosterone and DHT during this phase are critical for the formation of male internal and external genitalia structures.[21] Three to 6 months after birth, an LH surge drives a second peak in testosterone levels. This phase facilitates growth of a normal

phallus, testicular descent, Sertoli cell proliferation and spermatogonial development.[22–24] However, the low level of expression of AR on Sertoli cells during the fetal and infantile testosterone surges may serve to induce a period of relative androgen insensitivity and preserve Sertoli cell proliferation to allow for pubertal spermatogenic development later in life.[25] During adolescence, hypothalamic GnRH stimulates a third peak in testosterone, which results in the development of secondary sexual characteristics of the male and other changes in body, behavioral and sexual function. These changes include growth of the phallus and scrotum, male hair growth pattern, bone growth and mineralization and closure of epiphyseal plate, increase in skeletal muscle mass, erythropoiesis, increase in very low density lipoprotein (VLDL) and low density lipoprotein (LDL) and decrease in high density lipoprotein (HDL), spermatogenesis, and acquisition of fertility potential and spontaneous erections. In addition, testosterone mediates brain function changes including libido, motivation, aggressiveness, and cognitive function.[26] Through adult life, testosterone levels remain elevated to maintain many of these changes; however, with aging, a gradual decline in testosterone may contribute to alterations in muscle mass, bone mineral density, cardiovascular risk, libido, cognition, fertility, and erections.[27,28]

Testosterone levels demonstrate a predictable circadian rhythm that is dependent on sleep–wake cycles. Plasma levels begin to increase

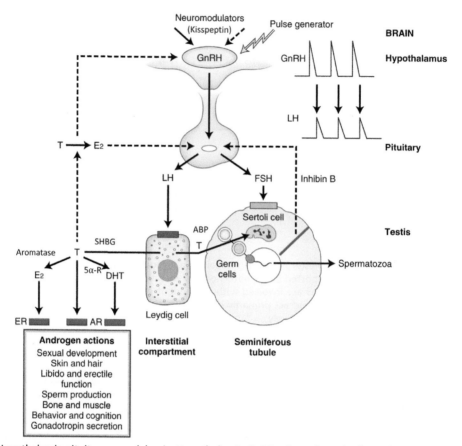

Fig. 2. Hypothalamic-pituitary-gonadal axis. Hypothalamic GnRH release into the hypophyseal portal system is driven by central neurotransmitter release in a pulsatile manner. The anterior pituitary is stimulated to produce LH and follicle-stimulating hormone. LH primarily acts on the Leydig cells in the testis to produce testosterone. Testosterone may then act on the Sertoli cells via androgen-binding protein within the seminiferous tubule to facilitate sperm production and maturation or enter the circulation bound to SHBG to affect distant target tissues. Peripherally, testosterone may be converted to DHT by 5α-reductase or estradiol by aromatase, which exert their own effects on target tissues. Testosterone and estradiol function as negative hypothalamic and pituitary feedback inhibitors. (*Adapted from*: Matsumoto AM, Anawalt BD. Testicular Disorders. In: Melmed S, ed. Williams Textbook of Endocrinology. 14th ed. Philadelphia: Elsevier; 2020:668-755; with permission.)

under the direction of LH at the onset of sleep and peak during the first 3 hours of sleep at the first rapid eye movement (REM) cycle. Testosterone remains at this level until waking, at which time it gradually declines while awake. There is also a superimposed ultradian rhythm with pulse increases every 90 minute throughout the day that reflects the pulsatile nature of LH release from the pituitary.[29] Overall, circadian rhythm disruptions do not seem to affect testosterone secretion and morning testosterone levels unless there is complete disruption of the sleep architecture preventing the initial increase in testosterone during the first REM cycle.[30,31] There has been substantial interest in assessing circannual variations in serum testosterone levels in men. The data are overall conflicting, with studies showing peak levels in winter months and nadir levels occurring during warm summer months, whereas other studies describe an opposite seasonal pattern or no variation at all. These differential findings may be attributed to differences in environments, temperatures, day–night patterns, timing of blood draws, and patient-specific factors.[32]

TESTOSTERONE REPLACEMENT THERAPY

Testosterone replacement therapy (TRT) is indicated for patients with primary hypogonadism, in which the condition originates in the testes, and secondary/hypogonadotropic hypogonadism, a disease of the hypothalamus or pituitary gland. The primary goal of TRT is to restore serum testosterone levels to within the mid-normal physiologic

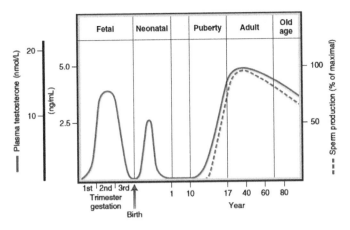

Fig. 3. Testosterone peaks in fetal, infant, and adolescent life. There are 3 peaks of serum testosterone in the lifetime of a man. The first in during fetal development and driven by maternal hCG and later by pituitary LH. The second occurs at 3 to 6 months of life and is responsible for penile growth, testicular descent, and Sertoli cell proliferation and development. Adolescence marks the third peak and gives rise secondary sexual characteristics and homeostatic mechanisms. (*From* Griffin JE, Wilson JD. The testis. In: Bondy PK, Rosenberg LE, eds. Metabolic Control and Disease, 8th ed. Philadelphia, PA: WB Saunders; 1980:1535–1578.)

range associated with the patient's age group, generally considered to be between 400 and 700 ng/dL and to improve symptoms in hypogonadal men. Because an estimated 2.4 million US men aged 40 to 69 years suffer from hypogonadism, the potential market for TRT is significant.[33] TRT efficacy and side effect profile are specific to each formulation, dose, and activity.

Soon after its synthesis in 1935, it became clear that, in reasonable doses, testosterone was not effective orally. We now know that the lack of oral effectiveness is due to the inactivation of testosterone by the first-pass effects in the liver and oral T administration would require extremely high doses. Currently, oral testosterone preparations are not available in the US due to low bioavailability along with gastrointestinal and liver adverse effects.[34] Fortunately, there are currently more than 30 different testosterone preparations to consider when choosing one for a patient, with different routes of delivery (topical gel, transdermal patch, buccal system [applied to upper gum or inner cheek], and injection), concentrations, and branded or generic choices.[33] Delivery and dosing information for formulations currently approved by the Food and Drug Administration (FDA) are highlighted in **Table 1**.

Subdermal testosterone pellets were the first effective formulation for androgen replacement therapy, developed in the 1940s, and pellets are still in use today.[35] Testosterone pellets are designed for consistent and prolonged release, and their application requires a small operation. Dosing varies on patient age and diagnosis, and generally vary from 75 to 450 mg implanted subdermally at 3 to 6 month intervals. Potential advantages of pellet usage include the guaranteed compliance, the steady levels of testosterone and lack of transference. Potential disadvantages include the risks of implantation, infection, and extrusion.[36]

In the 1980s, the first transdermal scrotal patches were found to be efficacious. This application allowed for maximal absorption through a thin-skinned area. Disadvantages included smaller skin surface area and application challenges (hair clipping). These scrotal patches have fallen out of favor and are no longer available.[37] Transdermal patches applied to the back, abdomen, upper arms, or thigh are effective and available but their efficacy is often limited by the lack of adherence or discontinuation due to skin blistering, pruritus, or irritation.[36]

In 2004, the intramuscular testosterone undecanoate preparation entered the market and led to widespread usage of TRT. Importantly, the intramuscular (IM) administration is associated with significant fluctuation in serum testosterone levels: following injection, the testosterone level peaks at supraphysiologic doses at 4 to 5 days and followed by slow decline to levels less than the lower limit of normal. These large fluctuations in serum testosterone levels over the cycle of IM TRT can result in significant mood swings or changes in libido. Although the United States FDA recommended starting dose for male hypogonadism is 50 to 400 mg IM every 2 to 4 weeks, many patients opt for shorter durations between IM TRT administration to minimize the testosterone fluctuation and to overcome the less than ideal kinetics of IM TRT. One additional disadvantage of IM TRT is the necessity for IM injection, which can be painful.[38]

Since 2002, several testosterone gels and liquids have been developed for transdermal TRT. The potential advantages of testosterone transdermal gels and liquids include ease of application, less skin irritation than patches, and more consistent serum testosterone levels than with IM TRT. However, due to the concern for testosterone gel or liquid being transferred to women and children who come into contact with a patient's skin after use, these

Table 1
Testosterone replacement therapies with Food and Drug Administration approval

Brand Name	Delivery System	Dose Delivery	Starting Dose	Dose Range
Androderm	Transdermal patch	2 or 4 mg patch	4 mg patch	2–6 mg
Androgel 1%	Transdermal gel	50 mg/packet 12.5 mg/pump	50 mg packet 4 pumps	50–100 mg
Androgel 1.62%		40.5 mg/packet 20.25 mg/pump	40.5 mg packet 2 pumps	20.25–81 mg
Testim		50 mg/tube	50 mg tube	50–100 mg
Fortesta		10 mg/pump	4 pumps	10–70 mg
Vogelxo		50 mg/tube 50 mg/packet 12.25 mg/pump	50 mg tube 50 mg packet 4 pumps	50–100 mg
Axiron	Transdermal lotion	30 mg/pump	2 pumps	30–120 mg
Striant	Buccal	30 mg/patch	1 patch Q12H	30 mg
Natesto	Nasal gel	11 mg/pump	1 pump per nostril Q8H	11 mg
Multiple	IM testosterone cypionate	IM injection	100 mg	50–200 mg every 7–14 d
Multiple	IM testosterone enanthate		100 mg	50–200 mg every 7–14 d
Aveed	IM testosterone undecanoate		750 mg at 0, 4, and then every 10 wk	750 mg
Testopel	Subcutaneous pellet	75 mg/pellet	10 pellets	6–12 pellets every 3–4 mo

formulations have received an FDA Boxed Warning. Patients should be reminded to wash their hands after application and to avoid skin contact with others. Recommended sites of application for these agents are areas that will be covered by clothing to minimize transfer.[36–38]

Additional FDA-approved TRT formulations include buccal administration (side effects gum irritation, inflammation, or gingivitis), nasal gel (side effects headache, rhinorrhea, nosebleed, nasal discomfort, upper respiratory tract infection, sinusitis, bronchitis, and nasal scab).[36,38]

The decision on the best product choice should include patient preference, treatment burden, cost, and insurance coverage. Products may also need to be switched throughout TRT based on patient response, preference, and adverse effects. In all circumstances, the decisions should be an open dialog between the patient and clinician to allow for the most successful TRT regimen. In addition, testosterone levels in patients should be considered.[33]

ANDROGEN DEPRIVATION THERAPY

In 1941, Charles Huggins at the University of Chicago reported that testosterone was a growth factor and the driver of prostate cancer and that prostate cancer was sensitive to surgical castration. This study subsequently led to a Nobel Prize in Medicine in 1966 for Huggins and established prostate cancer as a hormonally sensitive disease.[39] Surgical castration with bilateral orchiectomy rapidly results in castrate levels of testosterone (within 48 hours); however, the adrenal synthesis of testosterone is not affected. Chemical castration has become the mainstay of androgen deprivation therapy (ADT), due to the potential reversibility and avoidance of body dysmorphia with surgical castration.

ADT can be achieved through either GnRH agonists or antagonists. GnRH agonists are associated with an initial LH (and testosterone) surge and rely on a negative feedback loop. Within 4 weeks of initiation of therapy, the testosterone levels become castrate but concerns about the initial testosterone flare and its consequences for patients with metastatic prostate cancer must be considered. To avoid the effects of the flare, GnRH agonists are often preceded by direct AR antagonists, which block the downstream target of the androgens. In contrast, GnRH antagonists block LH and consequently testosterone production resulting in castrate levels of testosterone within 3 days of treatment.[40–42] For more detailed understanding of ADT, please refer the review by Saad and Fizazi.[40]

Although GnRH agonists and antagonists can stop the testicles from making androgens, cells in other parts of the body, such as the adrenal glands, and prostate cancer cells themselves, can still make testosterone. Some drugs can block the formation of androgens made by these cells, including inhibitors of steps in cholesterol synthesis, such as cytochrome P450 (CYP-17) inhibitors and nonsteroidal azoles. In addition, competitive antagonists of AR effectively block testosterone binding and activation of its target receptor.[40]

Because androgens have significant roles in multiple physiologic processes, the side effect profile of ADT is significant. Common adverse effects include "hot flashes," development of gynecomastia, sexual dysfunction, bone loss and skeletal morbidity, anemia, cognitive effects, metabolic alterations (sarcopenia, weight gain, fat deposition, insulin resistance, and increased triglycerides).[43]

THE ANDROGEN RECEPTOR

In 1989, Tilley, Wilson, and McPhaul cloned the human AR at the University of Texas Southwestern and provided the first evidence that the AR was a transcriptional factor that could regulate its own expression in prostate cancer.[44] The AR shares homology within the steroid hormone receptors superfamily, including the receptors for progesterone, mineralocorticoids, and glucocorticoids. It is composed of 920 amino acids and includes 4 key domains: the ligand-binding domain (LBD), the DNA-binding domain (DBD), the hinge domain, and an N-terminal transcription regulation domain (NTD) (**Fig. 4**). The NTD is the most variable among steroid hormone receptors, whereas the DBD is the most highly conserved.[45,46]

Structurally, the transcriptional prowess of the AR is attributed to the AR NTD. The NTD comprises more than half of the protein (amino acids 1–537) and includes polyglutamine and polyglycine stretches that vary and regulate the activity of the AR. Indeed, the length of the polyglutamine stretch in the AR correlates inversely with AR transcriptional activity: the longer the polyglutamine stretch, the less potent the AR as a transcription factor. In Kennedy disease, the polyglutamine stretch includes more than 36 glutamines resulting in altered function of the AR. In contrast, in normal men the polyglutamine stretch includes 10 to 35 glutamines.[47] Finally, although the NTD of AR is

60% of the protein, it is intrinsically disordered, and no structural information is available for this domain, which increases the difficulty of potential therapeutic targeting of the AR NTD.[48]

The AR DBD (residues 559–624) is highly conserved and encodes for 2 zinc fingers that enable interaction of AR with specific motifs on the DNA called AR responsive elements (AREs). Genes with AREs in their promoter are classically regulated by AR DNA binding and transcriptional regulation.[49] Mutations in this domain—which consist mainly of single nucleotide substitutions—cause the DNA-binding/dimerization activity of the protein to be defective, leading to impaired or absent transcriptional activation by the AR and can lead to androgen insensitivity syndromes.[49]

The hinge region (amino acids 625–669) enables androgen-dependent conformational changes in the AR.[50] Finally, the LBD of AR (residues 670–920) encodes helical motifs that enable androgen binding. The liganded LBD undergoes a conformational change, enabling AR dimerization, cofactor recruitment, and nuclear translocation. Cross talk between the liganded AR LBD and AR-NTD is critical for AR activity.[51] AR LBD mutations explaining the molecular basis of androgen resistance syndromes were first described by Wilson and McPhaul in the early 1990s. AR LBD mutations are commonly seen in complete androgen insensitivity syndromes, where genotypic XY males exhibit various female phenotypic characteristics including female external genitalia, underdeveloped vagina, absence of prostate, epididymis, vas deferentia, seminal vesicles, absence of sexual hair growth, and gynecomastia development.[52]

The AR is a potent transcription factor. The classic pathway (**Fig. 5**) describes the process in which androgens exert their effect on protein synthesis, a mechanism that results in physiologic changes over hours to days. When circulating bioavailable testosterone reaches its target tissue, it diffuses through the cellular membrane and binds to the cytoplasmic AR. Chaperone proteins bound to the AR dissociate with this interaction and allow the testosterone–AR complex to translocate to the nucleus, where it binds to the AREs within the regulatory sites of target genes. Recruitment of coregulatory proteins to the promoters of hundreds of AR-regulated genes then results in androgen-directed gene transcription and protein synthesis. In prostate cancer cells, the AR is thought to regulate up 5% of the transcriptional output of the cell. A secreted serine protease, prostate-specific antigen (PSA), is one of the canonical AR-regulated genes, and its expression level is virtually pathognomonic of active AR

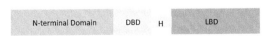

Fig. 4. AR. The AR is composed of a ligand-binding domain (LBD) at the C-terminus, which is separated from the DBD and N-terminal transcription domain by the Hinge region.

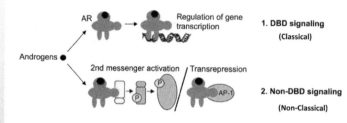

Fig. 5. Classical and nonclassical AR signal transduction. Androgens may affect changes in a target cell via the AR via classical and nonclassical mechanisms. In the classical mechanism, the AR ultimately regulates gene transcription and protein expression, producing an effect over hours to days. The nonclassical mechanism uses a second messenger signal transduction mechanism and produces an effect over seconds to minutes. (Rana Kesha, Davey Rachel A, Zajac Jeffrey D, Human androgen deficiency: insights gained from androgen receptor knockout mouse models, 2014, 16 (2), 169–177.)

signaling within the prostate. PSA expression also serves as an important biomarker of prostate cancer development and progression. Analyses of AR-mediated regulation of the PSA gene have revealed that ARE-bound AR recruits a plethora of coregulatory proteins, which play important roles in the initiation of transcription, as well as the fine-tuning of overall transcriptional output.[53,54] Large-scale gene expression profiling studies have indicated that approximately 1.5% to 5% of genes expressed in prostate cancer cells are directly or indirectly regulated by androgens. Similar to PSA, these AR-regulated genes have a profound impact on diverse cellular processes.[53,55]

Changes in expression levels (through AR amplification), point mutations, splice variants, and polymorphisms in the AR and alterations of coregulators or chaperone proteins may enable the AR to be active even without ligand binding and become independent of testosterone levels. Thus, AR signaling is active even when testosterone levels are castrate, leading to the development of castration-resistance when patients are being treated with ADT for advanced prostate cancer.[56–58]

A nonclassical pathway exists in which androgens produce a rapid effect on target tissues in seconds to minutes. These mechanisms involve both cell surface receptors and the activation of coregulators that lead to the activation of conventional signal transduction cascades using calcium, mitogen-activated protein kinase (MAPK), tyrosine kinases, and cyclic adenosine monophosphate (AMP). This nongenomic pathway can be found in brain, muscle, cardiovascular, prostate, immune, and Sertoli cells.[59,60] There is considerable debate about the relative contribution of the nongenomic and genomic pathways to differentiation and growth responses.

FDA-approved agents targeting the AR target the AR LBD. These include bicalutamide, enzalutamide, darolutamide, and apalutamide (**Table 2**). These agents bind to AR in the cytoplasm,

compete for testosterone binding to AR, and inhibit AR nuclear translocation, DNA binding, and transcriptional programming. Darolutamide is unique in that it seems to inhibit wild type and clinically relevant AR mutations that cause other antiandrogens to switch from antagonist to agonist. It also has lower penetration of the blood–brain barrier, resulting in reduced rates of CNS side effects.[61,62] Cells that are addicted to AR such as prostate cancer cells circumvent these agents by several methods, including AR gene amplification, AR LBD point mutations (that convert the AR antagonists to agonists), AR splice variants, and altered cofactor recruitment. It remains to be seen if agents that cause AR degradation can effectively overcome the cancer cell addiction to the AR.[63–65]

METABOLISM OF TESTOSTERONE (AROMATASE, 5α-REDUCTASE)

Circulating testosterone may exert its effects directly on target tissues and can also be converted to different steroid hormones. Aromatase adenosine monophosphate (CYP19) is an enzyme located especially in adipose tissue that converts testosterone to estradiol, and approximately 15% to 25% of circulating estradiol is produced in the testes by Leydig cells.[66] Estradiol promotes bone mineralization and epiphyseal plate closure, improves lipoprotein profiles and insulin sensitivity, and provides negative hypothalamic and pituitary feedback.[67,68]

DHT is formed from testosterone by the enzyme 5α-reductase (5AR), primarily within the skin and liver, and is 2.5 to 3.0 times more potent than testosterone. In prostate tissue, DHT is the primary ligand for the AR. There are 3 isoforms of 5AR. Type 1 is expressed most highly during puberty in the nongenital skin, contributing to sebum production. Type 2 is located in the genitourinary tract and other locations and is responsible for the development of the prostate and male external genitalia as well as the many changes that occur

Table 2
Agents targeting the androgen receptor

Agent	Brand Name	Class	Mechanism of Action	Side Effects
Biclutamide	Casodex	First-generation nonsteroidal antiandrogen	Competitive AR inhibition	Gynecomastia, breast pain, hot flushes, diarrhea
Enzlutamide	Xtandi	Second-generation nonsteroidal antiandrogen	Bind AR with high affinity Inhibit AR nuclear translocation	Fatigue, hypertension, hot flushes, falls, dizziness, nausea, risk of seizures
Apalutamide	Erleada		Inhibit AR DNA binding Inhibit coactivator recruitment	Fatigue, hypertension, rash, diarrhea, nausea, falls, hot flush, peripheral edema
Darolutamide	Nubeqa			Fatigue, nausea, extremity pain, rash, cardiovascular events

during the testosterone peak of puberty.[69] Overexpression of isoform 2 may be associated with the progression of benign prostatic hypertrophy (BPH) and lower urinary tract symptoms, whereas overexpression of isoform 1 within the prostate may be associated with prostatic adenocarcinoma.[70] Type 3 has been shown to be overexpressed in hormone-resistant prostate cancer cells.[71] Conversion of testosterone to DHT within the prostate results in intraprostatic levels of DHT that are 10 times higher than that of plasma, highlighting the autocrine and paracrine function of DHT within the prostate.[72,73] The key discovery was made at the University of Texas Southwestern in the 1960s by Bruchovsky and Wilson who discovered 5AR and its importance in converting testosterone to 5α-DHT as the primary hormone associated with prostatic growth.[74] Wilson went on to show that androgens are involved in every aspect of prostate development, growth, and function. Wenderoth and Wilson then showed that a 5AR inhibitor blocked the prostatic growth. These findings have been translated to widespread use of 5AR inhibitors in patients with BPH.[75]

SUMMARY

Testosterone and its steroid metabolite hormones play an exceedingly important role in the development of male sexual characteristics and function and in the homeostasis of numerous organ systems throughout the life cycle. Although the endocrine products of the testis created curiosity and excitement among early physiologists and physicians as a wondrous curative agent for everything from loss of strength, cognition and vitality to bowel and bladder habits, little was known regarding its production, mechanism of action and metabolism at that time. Present-day investigators have established the HPG axis as a tightly controlled feedback mechanism designed to strictly control homeostasis and have made great strides in characterization of the AR and its implications in normal physiologic as well as pathologic processes.

FUNDING

This article was made possible by funding to GVR from the Simmons Cancer Center at UT Southwestern for the Prostate Cancer Program, the Mimi and John Cole Prostate Cancer Fund, the Wilson Foundation and the Department of Defense Grants W81XWH-17-1-0674, W81XWH-19-1-0363, and W81XWH-21-1-0687.

CLINICS CARE POINTS

- Testosterone is a critical hormone in the development and maintenance of male characteristics and health.
- Testosterone levels predictably follow a normal lifetime and circadian pattern that should be considered during evaluation and management of hypogonadism.
- There are many options and delivery modalities for testosterone replacement therapy, each with their own profile and strengths and weaknesses.

- Androgen-deprivation therapy is a mainstay in the management of advanced prostate cancer. Clinicians treating patients in this setting should be familiar with the indications and side effects of each agent, particularly as the number of options and their applications expand.

DISCLOSURE

Nothing to disclose.

REFERENCES

1. Rostom M, Ramasamy R, Kohn TP. History of testosterone therapy through the ages. Int J Impot Res 2022. https://doi.org/10.1038/s41443-021-00493-w.
2. Brinkmann AO. Molecular Mechanisms of Androgen Action – A Historical Perspective. In: Saatcioglu F, editor. Androgen action - methods and Protocols. New York: Springer; 2011. p. 3–24.
3. Nieschlag E, Nieschlag S. Testosterone deficiency: a historical perspective. Asian J Androl 2014;16(2):161–8.
4. Brown-Sequard CE. The effects produced on man by subcutaneous injections of a liquid obtained from the testicles of animals. Lancet 1889;134(3438):105–7.
5. Cussons AJ, Bhagat CI, Fletcher SJ, et al. Brown-Séquard revisited: a lesson from history on the placebo effect of androgen treatment. Med J Aust 2002;177(11–12):678–9.
6. Rao PK, Boulet SL, Mehta A, et al. Trends in Testosterone Replacement Therapy Use from 2003 to 2013 among Reproductive-Age Men in the United States. J Urol 2017;197(4):1121–6.
7. Zhou CK, Advani S, Chaloux M, et al. Trends and Patterns of Testosterone Therapy among U.S. Male Medicare Beneficiaries, 1999 to 2014. J Urol 2020;203(6):1184–90.
8. Anawalt BD, Braunstein GD. Testes. In: Gardner DG, Shoback D, editors. Greenspan's Basic and Clinical Endocrinology, 10e. New York, NY: McGraw-Hill Education; 2017.
9. White BA, Harrison JR, Mehlmann LM. The Male Reproductive System. In: Endocrine and reproductive Physiology. St. Louis: Elsevier; 2019. p. 186–203.
10. Zirkin BR, Papadopoulos V. Leydig cells: formation, function, and regulation. Biol Reprod 2018;99(1):101–11.
11. Hammond GL, Ruokonen A, Kontturi M, et al. The simultaneous radioimmunoassay of seven steroids in human spermatic and peripheral venous blood. J Clin Endocrinology Metab 1977;45(1):16–24.
12. Skorupskaite K, George JT, Anderson RA. The kisspeptin-GnRH pathway in human reproductive health and disease. Hum Reprod Update 2014;20(4):485–500.
13. Harter CJL, Kavanagh GS, Smith JT. The role of kisspeptin neurons in reproduction and metabolism. J Endocrinol 2018;238(3):R173–83.
14. Kaprara A, Huhtaniemi IT. The hypothalamus-pituitary-gonad axis: Tales of mice and men. Metabolism 2018;86:3–17.
15. Handa RJ, Weiser MJ. Gonadal steroid hormones and the hypothalamo-pituitary-adrenal axis. Front Neuroendocrinol 2014;35(2):197–220.
16. Matsumoto AM, Anawalt BD. Testicular Disorders. In: Melmed S, editor. Williams Textbook of endocrinology. 14th edition. Philadelphia: Elsevier; 2020. p. 668–755.
17. Munell F, Suarez-Quian CA, Selva DM, et al. Androgen-binding protein and reproduction: where do we stand? J Androl 2002;23(5):598–609.
18. Keevil BG, Adaway J. Assessment of free testosterone concentration. J Steroid Biochem Mol Biol 2019;190:207–11.
19. Wan Q, Xie Y, Zhou Y, et al. Research progress on the relationship between sex hormone-binding globulin and male reproductive system diseases. Andrologia 2021;53(1):e13893.
20. Boeri L, Capogrosso P, Cazzaniga W, et al. SHBG levels in primary infertile men: a critical interpretation in clinical practice. Endocr Connect 2020;9(7):658–66.
21. Biason-Lauber A. Control of sex development. Best Pract Res Clin Endocrinol Metab 2010;24(2):163–86.
22. Rey RA. Mini-puberty and true puberty: differences in testicular function. Ann Endocrinol (Paris) 2014;75(2):58–63.
23. Edelsztein NY, Rey RA. Importance of the Androgen Receptor Signaling in Gene Transactivation and Transrepression for Pubertal Maturation of the Testis. Cells 2019;8(8).
24. Kuiri-Hanninen T, Sankilampi U, Dunkel L. Activation of the hypothalamic-pituitary-gonadal axis in infancy: minipuberty. Horm Res Paediatr 2014;82(2):73–80.
25. Rey RA, Musse M, Venara M, et al. Ontogeny of the androgen receptor expression in the fetal and postnatal testis: its relevance on Sertoli cell maturation and the onset of adult spermatogenesis. Microsc Res Tech 2009;72(11):787–95.
26. Rey RA. The Role of Androgen Signaling in Male Sexual Development at Puberty. Endocrinology 2021;162(2).
27. Kloner RA, Carson C 3rd, Dobs A, et al. Testosterone and Cardiovascular Disease. J Am Coll Cardiol 2016;67(5):545–57.
28. Blaya R, Blaya P, Rhoden L, et al. Low Testosterone Levels and Metabolic Syndrome in Aging Male. Curr Pharm Des 2017;23(30):4470–4.

29. Stamatiades GA, Kaiser UB. Gonadotropin regulation by pulsatile GnRH: Signaling and gene expression. Mol Cell Endocrinol 2018;463:131–41.

30. Wittert G. The relationship between sleep disorders and testosterone in men. Asian J Androl 2014;16(2):262–5.

31. Wittert G. The relationship between sleep disorders and testosterone. Curr Opin Endocrinol Diabetes Obes 2014;21(3):239–43.

32. Smith RP, Coward RM, Kovac JR, et al. The evidence for seasonal variations of testosterone in men. Maturitas 2013;74(3):208–12.

33. Mulhall JP, Trost LW, Brannigan RE, et al. Evaluation and Management of Testosterone Deficiency: AUA Guideline. J Urol 2018;200(2):423–32.

34. Murray-Lyon IM, Westaby D, Paradinas F. Hepatic complications of androgen therapy. Gastroenterology 1977;73(6):1461.

35. Deansley R, Parkes AS. Further experiments on the administration of hormones by the subcutaneous implantation of tablets. Lancet 1938;2:606–9.

36. Barbonetti A, D'Andrea S, Francavilla S. Testosterone replacement therapy. Andrology 2020;8(6):1551–66.

37. Gooren LJ, Bunck MC. Transdermal testosterone delivery: testosterone patch and gel. World J Urol 2003;21(5):316–9.

38. Wang C, Swerdloff RS. Testosterone Replacement Therapy in Hypogonadal Men. Endocrinol Metab Clin North Am 2022;51(1):77–98.

39. Huggins C, Hodges CV. The effect of castration, of estrogen and androgen injection on serum phosphatases in metastatic carcinoma of the prostate. Cancer Res 1941;1:293–7.

40. Saad F, Fizazi K. Androgen Deprivation Therapy and Secondary Hormone Therapy in the Management of Hormone-sensitive and Castration-resistant Prostate Cancer. Urology 2015;86(5):852–61.

41. Lowrance WT, Breau RH, Chou R, et al. Advanced Prostate Cancer: AUA/ASTRO/SUO Guideline PART I. J Urol 2021;205(1):14–21.

42. Lowrance WT, Breau RH, Chou R, et al. Advanced Prostate Cancer: AUA/ASTRO/SUO Guideline PART II. J Urol 2021;205(1):22–9.

43. Magee DE, Singal RK. Androgen deprivation therapy: indications, methods of utilization, side effects, and their management. Can J Urol 2020;27:11–6.

44. Tilley WD, Marcelli M, Wilson JD, et al. Characterization and expression of a cDNA encoding the human androgen receptor. Proc Natl Acad Sci USA 1989;86(1):327–31.

45. Davey RA, Grossman M. Androgen Receptor Structure, Function and Biology: From Bench to Bedside. Clin Biochem Rev 2016;37(1).

46. MacLean HE, Warne GL, Zajac JD. Localization of Functional Domains in the Androgen Receptor. J Steroid Biochem Mol Biol 1997;62(4):233–42.

47. Palazzolo I, Gliozzi A, Rusmini P, et al. The role of the polyglutamine tract in androgen receptor. J Steroid Biochem Mol Biol 2008;108(3–5):245–53.

48. Sadar MD. Discovery of drugs that directly target the intrinsically disordered region of the androgen receptor. Expert Opin Drug Discov 2020;15(5):551–60.

49. Geserick C, Meyer HA, Haendler B. The role of DNA response elements as allosteric modulators of steroid receptor function. Mol Cell Endocrinol 2005;236(1–2):1–7.

50. Clinckemalie L, Vanderschueren D, Boonen S, et al. The hinge region in androgen receptor control. Mol Cell Endocrinol 2012;358(1):1–8.

51. Steketee K, Berrevoets CA, Dubbink HJ, et al. Amino acids 3-13 and amino acids in and flanking the 23FxxLF27 motif modulate the interaction between the N-terminal and ligand-binding domain of the androgen receptor. Eur J Biochem 2002;269(23):5780–91.

52. McPhaul MJ, Marcelli M, Zoppi S, et al. Mutations in the ligand-binding domain of the androgen receptor gene cluster in two regions of the gene. J Clin Invest 1992;90(5):2097–101.

53. Agoulnik IU, Weigel NL. Androgen receptor action in hormone-dependent and recurrent prostate cancer. J Cell Biochem 2006;99(2):362–72.

54. Kim J, Coetzee GA. Prostate specific antigen gene regulation by androgen receptor. J Cell Biochem 2004;93(2):233–41.

55. Culig Z, Santer FR. Androgen receptor signaling in prostate cancer. Cancer Metastasis Rev 2014;33(2–3):413–27.

56. Koochekpour S. Androgen receptor signaling and mutations in prostate cancer. Asian J Androl 2010;12(5):639–57.

57. Armstrong CM, Gao AC. Dysregulated androgen synthesis and anti-androgen resistance in advanced prostate cancer. Am J Clin Exp Urol 2021;9(4):292–300.

58. Yuan X, Cai C, Chen S, et al. Androgen receptor functions in castration-resistant prostate cancer and mechanisms of resistance to new agents targeting the androgen axis. Oncogene 2014;33(22):2815–25.

59. Cooke PS, Walker WH. Nonclassical androgen and estrogen signaling is essential for normal spermatogenesis. Semin Cell Dev Biol 2022;121:71–81.

60. Deng Q, Zhang Z, Wu Y, et al. Non-Genomic Action of Androgens is Mediated by Rapid Phosphorylation and Regulation of Androgen Receptor Trafficking. Cell Physiol Biochem 2017;43(1):223–36.

61. Darolutamide Aragon-Ching JB. a novel androgen-signaling agent in nonmetastatic castration-resistant prostate cancer. Asian J Androl 2020;22(1):76–8.

62. Rice MA, Malhotra SV, Stoyanova T. Second-Generation Antiandrogens: From Discovery to Standard of Care in Castration Resistant Prostate Cancer. Front Oncol 2019;9:801.

63. Schmidt KT, Huitema ADR, Chau CH, et al. Resistance to second-generation androgen receptor antagonists in prostate cancer. Nat Rev Urol 2021; 18(4):209–26.

64. Rajaram P, Rivera A, Muthima K, et al. Second-Generation Androgen Receptor Antagonists as Hormonal Therapeutics for Three Forms of Prostate Cancer. Molecules 2020;25(10).

65. Rathkopf D, Scher HI. Androgen Receptor Antagonists in Castration-Resistant Prostate Cancer. Cancer J 2013;19(1):43–9.

66. Cooke PS, Nanjappa MK, Ko C, et al. Estrogens in Male Physiology. Physiol Rev 2017;97(3): 995–1043.

67. Schulster M, Bernie AM, Ramasamy R. The role of estradiol in male reproductive function. Asian J Androl 2016;18(3):435–40.

68. Lo EM, Rodriguez KM, Pastuszak AW, et al. Alternatives to Testosterone Therapy: A Review. Sex Med Rev 2018;6(1):106–13.

69. Fullhase C, Schneider MP. 5-Alpha-Reductase Inhibitors and Combination Therapy. Urol Clin North Am 2016;43(3):325–36.

70. Wang K, Fan DD, Jin S, et al. Differential expression of 5-alpha reductase isozymes in the prostate and its clinical implications. Asian J Androl 2014;16(2): 274–9.

71. Uemura M, Tamura K, Chung S, et al. Novel 5 alpha-steroid reductase (SRD5A3, type-3) is overexpressed in hormone-refractory prostate cancer. Cancer Sci 2008;99(1):81–6.

72. Swerdloff RS, Dudley RE, Page ST, et al. Dihydrotestosterone: Biochemistry, Physiology, and Clinical Implications of Elevated Blood Levels. Endocr Rev 2017;38(3):220–54.

73. van der Sluis TM, Meuleman EJ, van Moorselaar RJ, et al. Intraprostatic testosterone and dihydrotestosterone. Part II: concentrations after androgen hormonal manipulation in men with benign prostatic hyperplasia and prostate cancer. BJU Int 2012; 109(2):183–8.

74. Bruchovsky N, Wilson JD. The conversion of testosterone to 5-alpha-androstan-17-beta-ol-3-one by rat prostate in vivo and in vitro. J Biol Chem 1968;243: 2012–21.

75. Wenderoth UK, George FW, Wilson JD. The effect of a 5 alpha-reductase inhibitor on androgen-mediated growth of the dog prostate. Endocrinology 1983; 113:569–73.

Molecular Mechanisms of Castrate-Resistant Prostate Cancer

Srinath Kotamarti, MD[a], Andrew J. Armstrong, MD[a,b], Thomas J. Polascik, MD[a], Judd W. Moul, MD[a,*]

KEYWORDS

- Prostate cancer • Castrate resistance • Therapeutic resistance • Androgen receptor

KEY POINTS

- Despite therapeutic advances, most patients with castrate-resistant prostate cancer will experience primary or secondary resistance.
- Several androgen receptor (AR)-related and AR-independent resistance pathways have been identified.
- Research has spurred the development of novel biomarkers and molecularly targeted treatments.

INTRODUCTION

Advanced prostate cancer (PCa) treatment classically has centered on androgen modulation, with androgen deprivation therapy (ADT) as the standard of care for greater than 50 years.[1] Castrate levels of testosterone decrease cancer proliferation and induce cellular apoptosis.[2] However, over time, certain cells adapt and resume proliferation with an associated rise in prostate-specific antigen (PSA) leading to castrate-resistance (CR) with/without metastases development.[1] In the past decade, newer androgen receptor (AR) signaling inhibitors (ARSIs) have been added to the armamentarium including abiraterone, enzalutamide, apalutamide, and darolutamide. Still, many patients have primary resistance, and most will experience secondary or cross-resistance over several years, with resistance mechanisms still being understood (**Fig. 1**).[3–6] Although contemporary progression to CR PCa (CRPC) typically happens after ARSI treatment, CRPC often is not independent of AR activation and still relies on related signaling pathways[7]; however, approximately 20% to 30% of patients with metastatic CRPC (mCRPC) post-ARSI will show AR-independence and AR expression-loss.[8,9] Importantly, mechanisms contributing toward CR development likely also persist into CRPC as patients progress through therapies. Herein, we discuss the molecular mechanisms allowing for therapeutic impedance in CRPC, considered to be either AR-related or AR-unrelated.

ANDROGEN RECEPTOR-RELATED MECHANISMS

Located at Xq11 to 12, AR is a steroid hormone nuclear receptor and transcription factor.[10] Through various mechanisms, AR function can be modulated to limit/negate therapeutic interventions in CRPC (**Fig. 2**, **Table 1**).

Androgen Receptor Splice Variants

AR splice variants (AR-Vs) are truncated AR proteins prone to persistent activation.[11] AR-Vs can be produced through genomic structural rearrangements (GSRs) during ADT, altered mRNA-splicing, or high transcriptional rates of the full-length AR, itself.[12] These variants lack the

[a] Division of Urology, Duke Cancer Institute, 20 Duke Medicine Circle, Durham, NC 27710, USA; [b] Division of Medical Oncology, Duke Cancer Institute, 20 Duke Medicine Circle, Durham, NC 27710, USA
* Corresponding author. Division of Urology, Duke University Medical Center, Room 1562 Blue Zone, Duke South, Durham, NC 27710.
E-mail address: judd.moul@duke.edu

Urol Clin N Am 49 (2022) 615–626
https://doi.org/10.1016/j.ucl.2022.07.005
0094-0143/22/© 2022 Elsevier Inc. All rights reserved.

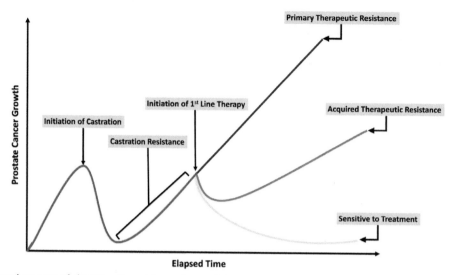

Fig. 1. Development of therapeutic resistance in prostate cancer.

C-terminal ligand-binding domain (LBD), keeping the transactivating N-terminal domain (**Fig. 3**).[13] Unable to bind ligand, aberrant ARs are constitutively-activated transcription factors.[11] Of several identified AR-Vs, AR-V7 is a key variant with a known protein product and analytically/clinically validated biomarker for detection in circulating tumor cells (CTCs). It has been shown to have increased expression within CRPC and high rate of ligand-independent activity, enhanced further by factors including HOXB13.[1,14] One study showed AR-V7+ mCRPC patients starting an ARSI to have worse PSA response than AR-V7− patients for enzalutamide and abiraterone (0% vs 53% and 0% vs 68%, respectively).[7] These patients also had worse overall survival (OS) for both ARSIs (median 5.5 months vs not reached, and 10.6 months vs not reached, respectively), and inferior PSA and clinical/radiographic progression-free survival (PFS).[7] In another study of men with progressive mCRPC evaluating AR-V7 status to predict OS after ARSI or taxane chemotherapy, AR-V7 positivity in high-risk patients was associated with shorter median OS in

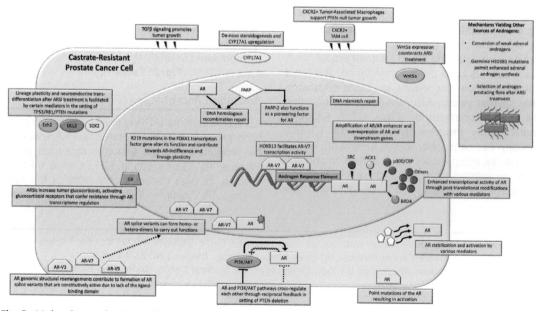

Fig. 2. Molecular mechanisms of castrate-resistant prostate cancer.

Table 1
Mentioned mechanisms of therapeutic resistance in CRPC

Mechanisms of Resistance Related to AR-Targeted Therapy

AR splice variants	Truncated proteins with a lack of ligand-binding domain that are constitutively active, forming homo- or hetero-dimers to carry out transcription activities Formed by mechanisms including genomic structural rearrangements AR variant-7 transcription activity is facilitated by factors including HOXB13
Amplification of AR genes and related enhancers	Associated with AR signaling-inhibitor resistance and worse clinical outcomes
Mutations of the AR	Point mutations are associated with conformal changes, including within the ligand-binding domain, conferring therapeutic resistance
AR stabilization	Mediated through factors including HER2/HER3 activation or SPOP degradation
Enhanced AR transcriptional activity	Mediated through post-translational modifications including phosphorylation, acetylation, and methylation with various mediators including SRC, ACK1, p300/CBP, BRD4, and others Aside from regulating DNA homologous recombination repair, PARP-2 also functions as a pioneering factor for AR through interactions with FOXA1
Impact of the microbiome	Selection of androgen-producing flora after AR signaling-inhibitor treatment including *Ruminococcus* and *Clostridiales bacterium*
Enhanced steroidogenesis and expression of CYP17A1	Continued androgen production may occur from the conversion of weak adrenal androgens, germline HSD3B1 mutations that permit enhanced adrenal androgen synthesis, or de-novo creation from cholesterol AR-targeted therapy may select for cells prone to increased expression of genes encoding for enzymes involved in steroidogenesis including CYP17A1, AKR1C3, and HSD3B2
Alternate AR-related pathways of signal transduction	PI3K/AKT and AR pathways cross-regulate each other through reciprocal feedback in the setting of PTEN-loss CXCR2+ tumor-associated macrophages support PTEN-null tumor growth Androgen-targeted therapy increases tumor glucocorticoids, activating glucocorticoid receptors that regulate the AR transcriptome
Neuroendocrine prostate cancer trans-differentiation and lineage plasticity	Selection of AR-independent cells with a progressive phenotype Facilitated by certain mediators such as Ezh2, DLL3, and SOX2 in the setting of TP53/RB1/PTEN mutations R219 mutations in the FOXA1 gene alter its transcription factor function and contribute toward lineage-switching

Mechanisms of Resistance Unrelated to AR-Targeted Therapy	
Homologous repair-deficient genes	Although AR plays a role in DNA repair regulation, such gene alterations are considered a predictor of AR-targeted therapeutic resistance DNA homologous repair deficiency is suggested to correlate with metastatic CRPC progression and has led to the incorporation of PARP-inhibitors
DNA mismatch repair gene mutations	Along with high microsatellite instability, such mutations are the target of PD-1 inhibition
Wnt pathway and Wnt5a expression	Wnt5a expression has been shown to counteract AR-target treatment
Transforming growth factor-β signaling	TGFβ signaling promotes tumor growth in CRPC

Abbreviations: AR, androgen receptor; CRPC, castrate-resistant prostate cancer.

those receiving ARSI (5.6 vs 14.3 months, $P = .03$), showing the prognostic value of CTC-detected AR-V7.[15] The PROPHECY trial expanded on this concept, analyzing 118 men with high-risk mCRPC initiating abiraterone or enzalutamide using two different blood assays.[16] AR-V7 positivity was associated with both shorter PFS and OS using either assay, suggesting the need for non-ARSIs in this subset.[16] Interestingly, patients undergoing subsequent taxane chemotherapy did not experience inferior PFS/OS and therefore may still derive benefit in cases of AR-V7 positivity.[7,17,18] AR-V7 further offers promise as a biomarker of cross-resistance between ARSIs in approximately 20% of patients; however, it currently does not provide insight when lack of response to chemotherapy occurs.[1] Thus, AR-V7 analysis can likely be considered clinically in the decision-making for therapies including and beyond second-line after prior ARSI treatment.[10] Still, AR-Vs explain only a minority of ARSI cross-resistance.

Amplification of Androgen Receptor Genes/Enhancers

Increased AR expression has been implicated with ARSI-resistance, as Xq11-q12 amplifications may reflect AR gene overexpression and lead to AR-targeting therapeutic impedance.[10] Overexpression can occur from AR gene amplification, found in up to 50% of patients with mCRPC in the second-line setting, compared with only 10% to 15% in treatment-naïve patients.[19] One study suggested that up to 80% of patients with CRPC show an elevated AR gene copy number, with 30% showing high-level amplification.[20] In a multicohort analysis of patients with mCRPC receiving first-line abiraterone or enzalutamide, those with a

plasma AR copy-number [3] 1.92 were associated with shorter PFS and OS, along with a shorter response to prior primary ADT.[21] In another study, AR amplification in plasma cell-free DNA (cfDNA) showed a similar prognostic value to CTCs [3] 5 in mCRPC, although both featured similarly weak areas under the curve values (0.66 and 0.68, respectively).[22] Activation and amplification of AR-related enhancers has also been implicated in mCRPC progression, with cases of increased expression compared with the AR gene.[23] Increased enhancer copy-number was shown to upregulate proliferation and confer enzalutamide resistance.[23] Another study showed cfDNA-based enhancer amplification is present in 40% of patients with mPCa treated with an ARSI and associated with worse 6-month PFS and OS than those without amplification (30% vs 71%, $P = .0002$, and 59% vs 100%, $P = .0015$, respectively).[24] Ongoing clinical trials including NCT03700099 and NCT02922218 will clarify if AR overexpression can be used in treatment selection.[10] Thus, ctDNA detection of AR gain is prognostic, but may not be sufficiently predictive to guide mCRPC treatment decision-making.

Mutations of the Androgen Receptor

CRPC is increasingly associated with gene-level aberrations including AR LBD point mutations and gene-amplification in up to 10% to 30% of patients with CR undergoing ARSIs.[20] Acquired AR mutations can also occur through continued treatment with AR antagonists.[25] AR exon-8 alterations may cause changes within LBD steroid-binding pockets, leading AR antagonists to act as agonists.[26] Preclinical studies previously showed that AR F876 L missense mutation in the LBD modifies AR antagonists into partial agonists,

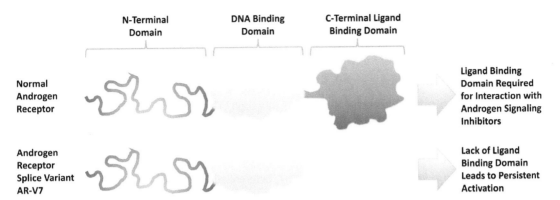

Fig. 3. Androgen receptor splice variant-7 (AR-V7).

conferring therapeutic resistance.[27] Another study analyzed DNA extracted from 62 mCRPC men progressing post-ARSIs, finding missense exon-8 mutations in 18% of patients.[19] Carreira and colleagues[28] sequenced the AR-coding exons in patients receiving exogenous glucocorticoids, finding AR LBD mutations at AR-L702H, AR-H875Y, and AR-T878 A; mutations featured a temporal relationship between their emergence and development of resistance to ARSIs administered with glucocorticoids. Furthermore, in mCRPC, gene alterations rendering the AR responsive to progesterone have been associated with abiraterone resistance.[29] CYP17A1 inhibition was shown to increase intracellular progesterone, influencing gene expression and subsequent AR-mediated resistance in cancers with T877 A or T878 A mutations.[29,30]

Androgen Receptor Stabilization

AR stabilization in CRPC is thought to be associated with poorer outcomes.[31] Longer AR half-life under lower androgen levels once stabilized may serve as a resistance mediator through hypersensitizing the receptor to its ligand.[25] Proteins including HER2 and HER3 have been shown to promote AR stabilization in CR.[25,32] Zhang and colleagues[33] recently further associated HER3-activation as a means through which neuregulin-1 (NRG1), an epidermal growth factor gene, promotes resistance. SPOP, an E3 ubiquitin ligase adaptor serving as a PCa-inhibitor that is altered in 15% of cases, also affects AR stabilization; specifically, AR stabilization occurs with SPOP degradation, which is mediated through LIM kinase-2 phosphorylation.[34] SPOP mutations are associated with improved responses and survival with hormonal therapy in advanced PCa and are de-enriched in mCRPC.[35]

Enhanced Androgen Receptor Transcriptional Activity

Post-translational AR modifications can enhance AR transcriptional activity at lower androgen levels.[25] Such alterations, including phosphorylation (through ACK1, PIM-1, SRC, etc.), acetylation (through ARD1, p300, etc.), and methylation (through DOT1L, Set9, PRMT5, etc.) are associated with increased AR function,[36] contributing to AR reactivation in the CR state and subsequent ARSI-resistance.[37] Increased tyrosine phosphorylation in CRPC is mediated by kinases like SRC and ACK1 that are increased at low androgen levels.[25] Dasatinib, a multikinase inhibitor blocking the SRC kinase family, was evaluated in a phase-3 mCRPC trial with no OS advantage versus docetaxel found.[38] Interleukin-6, shown to mediate PCa progression through upregulation of translation initiation factor eIF4a (TIF2), was also evaluated in CRPC phase-2 trials that showed minimal clinical activity.[39,40] The poly(ADP-ribose) polymerase (PARP) enzyme family, specifically PARP-2, aside from its role in DNA damage repair, is also a pioneering factor along with FOXA1 for AR activity.[41] Numerous other oncogenic pathways have also been described, including HER2/3, IGFR, p38, PI3K/AKT, and many more. BRD4 protein, for example, regulates transcription through AR-binding and has been implicated as a therapeutic target.[36] In addition, AR transcriptional coactivators p300 and CBP are enhanced after ARSI treatment through CREB1 phosphorylation and have been implicated in CRPC as therapeutic resistance mediators[42]; these histone acetyltransferase proteins have recently been studied as treatment targets.[43]

Impact of the Microbiome

Composed of the microorganisms living symbiotically within the host, the microbiota and its impact on PCa have been evaluated. Pernigoni and colleagues[44] evaluated the role of gut micriobiota on host hormone metabolism. ARSI treatment was found to be associated with the emergence of gut species that could generate androgens from precursors, and *Ruminococcus* and *Clostridiales bacterium* identification in patients with CRPC was linked with poor clinical outcomes.[44] The authors further showed the impact of fecal microbiota transplantation (FMT), with CRPC FMT transitioning mice with PCa to CRPC, and hormone-sensitive PCa (HSPCa) FMT controlling tumor growth.[44]

Enhanced Steroidogenesis and Expression of CYP17A1

CR transition after ARSIs fails still allows for continued androgen-related impact. Increased intratumoral production of testosterone and dihydrotestosterone from weak androgens synthesized by the adrenal glands, and possible de-novo creation from cholesterol, may reactivate the AR.[45] Indeed, HSD3B1 germline mutations have been linked to an "adrenal-permissive" HSD3B1(1245C) allele that allows for dihydrotestosterone synthesis and impaired ARSI response in mCRPC.[46] Although abiraterone potently inhibits CYP17A1, numerous genes involved in androgen biosynthesis are upregulated posttreatment.[47] Abiraterone may also select for cells prone to increased intratumoral CYP17A1 expression and subsequent androgen synthesis.[29] Other implicated enzymes that may be elevated include AKR1C3 and HSD3B2.[48,49]

Alternate Androgen Receptor-Related Pathways of Signal Transduction

Various other signal transduction pathways are associated with AR-related therapeutic resistance. NF-KB increases AR-V expression and is associated with androgen desensitization of PCa cells.[50] CRPC has also been associated to involve pathways including PI3K/AKT, which engages with AR in cross-regulation through reciprocal feedback in the setting of PTEN-deletion.[25,51] In the phase-3 IPATenttial150 trial evaluating ipatasertib (AKT-inhibitor) in mCRPC, ipatasertib/abiraterone combination showed improved radiographic PFS (rPFS) versus placebo/abiraterone (18.5 months vs 16.5 months, $P = .034$) in mCRPC patients with PTEN-loss; however, this was not appreciated in the intention-to-treat population.[52] OS was also not improved, suggesting additional parallel processes are activated during AR/AKT-inhibition in this setting.[52]

Further alternate pathways involve tumor microenvironment and stromal signaling that creates a paracrine effect on CRPC development. CXCR2 is a chemokine receptor expressed in tumor-associated macrophages (TAMs); CXCR2+ TAMs sustain tumor growth in PTEN-null cells through T-cell suppression and vessel formation.[53] Conversely, CXCR2 blockade is associated with TAM TNFa release, causing senescence and tumor inhibition.[53] CXCR2 has also been implicated in neuroendocrine PCa (NEPC) trans-differentiation through AR-expression loss, ARSI-resistance, and lineage plasticity; this mechanism has been successfully targeted through combined CXCR2/AR inhibition.[54]

Closely related to AR, the glucocorticosteroid receptor (GR) has also been implicated in enabling PCa cell survival despite ARSIs.[55] AR treatment induces glucocorticoid metabolism alterations, mediated through 11b-HSD, increasing tumor glucocorticoids, and therefore enabling GR signaling.[55] Mifepristone is a nonselective steroidal nuclear hormone antagonist capable of GR-antagonization that was recently assessed in a phase-1/2 CRPC trial with enzalutamide.[56] Although well-tolerated, the mifepristone/enzalutamide combination did not lead to PSA or PFS improvement.[56] As mifepristone can raise testosterone levels, more selective GR-modulators including relacorilant (NCT03674814) and exicorilant (NCT03437941) are being studied in phase-1 trials.[56]

Neuroendocrine Advanced Prostate Cancer Trans-differentiation and Lineage Plasticity

Post-ADT, PCa progression can also occur in an androgen-independent manner called NEPC trans-differentiation. Neuroendocrine tumor cells are less responsive to ADT, allowing for growth beyond adenocarcinomas.[10] Linked to NEPC trans-differentiation, lineage plasticity is also implicated, as a high-plasticity state occurs post-ARSI that induces stem-cell-like properties and shifts AR-dependent luminal epithelial cells to AR-independent basal cells, conferring a progressive phenotype.[57–60] Through lineage-switching, tumors develop ARSI-resistance and undergo both genetic/epigenetic divergent clonal evolution.[9,58,59] Although these cells often are without AR expression, in some patients AR expression can be retained despite AR transcriptional activity loss, causing low PSA production despite high-volume metastases.[9] This AR-independent growth leads to the CR state and is found in approximately 30% of men with lethal mCRPC at autopsy.[8,61] In fact, 32.1% of all

CRPC patients feature AR expression loss, with neuroendocrine trans-differentiation associated with half of these AR-indifferent tumors and approximately 10% to 15% of men developing AR-negative non-NEPC poorly-differentiated tumors; all are associated with poor prognosis.[8,61] Neuroendocrine differentiation has also been linked to markers like chromogranin-A and neuron-specific enolase, as well as a higher rate of loss-of-function mutations or deletions in critical tumor suppressor genes (TP53, RB1, and PTEN), which regulate lineage state, plasticity, and metastatic spread.[10,62] Alterations associated with neuroendocrine differentiation have been recently implicated in ARSI-resistance and, whereas not exclusive to NEPC, are highly enriched.[10] For example, R219 mutations in the FOXA1 transcription factor gene have been shown to alter its function, blocking luminal differentiation and contributing to AR-indifference and lineage plasticity.[63] A NEPC CTC assay has also been developed and shown this phenotype to be independently associated with worse OS (HR 3.8, 95% CI 1.2–12.3) in mCRPC men post-ARSIs.[64] Interestingly, ARSI-resistant NEPC can also develop without AR inhibition.[65]

Recent investigations have considered mechanisms involved in these processes as potential therapeutic targets. Considering N-myc, associated with NEPC progression, Beltran and colleagues[66] recently evaluated alisertib, an N-myc signaling inhibitor, in a phase-2 trial of 60 men with mPCa and features suggestive of neuroendocrine differentiation. Unfortunately, the primary endpoint of rPFS was unsuccessful; however, study is ongoing to identify more selective N-myc-inhibiting drugs.[66] Regarding transcription factor SOX2, Mu and colleagues[57] used PCa models to show lineage switch to AR-independence through the transition from luminal to basal-like cells. Although SOX2 is typically repressed by AR in PCa, enzalutamide treatment in the setting of TP53 and RB1 loss spurred the observed lineage plasticity mediated by SOX2, which could be undone with the restoration of TP53/RB1 and SOX2 inhibition.[57] Enhanced expression of epigenetic reprogramming factor Ezh2 has also been implicated in TP53/RB1 loss[59]; inhibition restored sensitivity to ARSI treatment in a preclinical model, and there are ongoing clinical trials for Ezh2 inhibitors such as Tazemetostat (NCT04179864).[60] DLL3 (delta-like protein 3) expression has also been correlated with NEPC and RB1 loss and has been targeted with anti-DLL3 antibody-drug conjugates in ongoing trials.[67]

ANDROGEN RECEPTOR-UNRELATED MECHANISMS

Alternative processes at work in advanced PCa have been discovered, each with potentially actionable targets (see **Table 1**). Defects in homologous recombination repair (HRR)-deficient genes occur in 20% to 25% of patients with mCRPC.[68] Although AR plays a role in DNA repair regulation, such gene alterations have been considered a predictor of ARSI resistance; however, they have been shown to be susceptible to PARP-inhibitors and possibly platinum-based treatments.[10,69] In the phase-3 PROfound trial, PARP-inhibitor olaparib in mCRPC patients with [3] one BRCA1/BRCA2/ATM alteration was associated with improved rPFS and OS compared with ARSI.[70] Preclinical models have also shown loss of both BRCA2 and RB1 to induce epithelial-mesenchymal transition.[71] Assessing the potential of a synergistic relationship between AR and PARP inhibition in mCRPC, preliminary data from a phase-2 trial of abiraterone ± olaparib suggested improved PFS irrespective of HRR-deficiency presence, which led to the phase-3 PROPEL and MAGNITUDE trials testing olaparib or niraparib with abiraterone in first-line mCRPC.[72,73] In PROPEL, olaparib plus abiraterone extended rPFS by 8 to 11 months over abiraterone alone, with significant benefits observed in HRR+ (HR 0.50) and HRR– mCRPC patients (HR 0.76).[72] In MAGNITUDE, a significant benefit was only observed in men harboring BRCA1/2 alterations (HR 0.5), suggesting that efficacy differences may exist between PARP-inhibitors or trial design variations may have contributed to the disparity in outcomes.[73] These results, if confirmed with longer-term survival data, suggest that DNA repair deficiency contributes strongly to mCRPC progression, and that this may be overcome through the early use of combined PARP/AR inhibition.

Germline mutations in DNA mismatch repair genes have been described in 0.6% of mCRPC men, although a hypermutated phenotype could exist in up to 12%.[74] Microsatellite instability-high (MSI-high) mCRPC is present in around 3% to 6% of patients. Pembrolizumab (anti-PD-1), now approved for cancers with defective DNA mismatch repair genes or MSI-high disease, may be an attractive treatment for such patients with progression post-ARSIs.[75,76]

Other relevant processes include the Wnt pathway and TGF-b inhibition. Chen and colleagues[77] identified the Wnt/b-catenin pathway as the most upregulated in mCRPC patients with enzalutamide resistance undergoing whole-genome and whole-transcriptome RNA sequencing. Miyamoto and colleagues[78] further showed noncanonical Wnt signaling in CTCs from patients with CRPC progressing through an ARSI, showing cellular Wnt5a expression's ability to counteract ARSI action. Regarding TGF-b signaling, galunisertib, a TGF-b receptor-I inhibitor, in combination with enzalutamide, suppressed PCa growth in a preclinical model ($P < .05$)[79]; this combination is currently being studied in a phase-2 trial, NCT02452008.

DISCUSSION

Advanced PCa is a complex process affected by adrenal, paracrine, and autocrine sources of androgen, as well as numerous mechanisms of persistent AR activation in the face of castration and AR-bypass mechanisms that develop over time. Numerous resistance mechanisms can be identified through clinical biomarkers including DNA genotyping, AR-V detection, tumor phenotyping of histologic transformation, and loss of AR-dependence. Disease course heterogeneity reflects the marked heterogeneity at the molecular level both within patients and between patients.[80,81] Indeed, initial and subsequent systemic therapies drive further tumor adaptations. Personalized treatment approach is required, depending on the unique combination of mechanisms used by the tumor at a given point in time. Suggested by early use of ARSI and docetaxel extending survival in mHSPCa, early combination approaches are more effective than waiting for resistance to occur. Ongoing studies of early combination trials of novel agents targeting PSMA, AR, DNA repair, metastasis-directed therapies, and tumor immune escape will test the utility of mCRPC prevention/delay strategies.

The role of genetic testing in advanced PCa management is ever-expanding. Well-studied resistance mechanisms have potential as biomarkers serving as treatment response predictors. AR-V7 represents one of possibly several clinically-validated prognostic and potentially predictive biomarkers; using nuclear protein or mRNA detection assays, it may be able to direct certain patients away from less effective second-line ARSIs, providing them more beneficial treatments earlier.[25] Several CTC-based AR-V7 assays are commercially available, although the Epic Sciences (Epic Sciences, San Diego, CA) assay is currently the only one Medicare-reimbursed.[25] Interest in this subject has also been evident through the growth of testing options. For example, FoundationOne CDx (Foundation Medicine, Cambridge, Massachusetts) is an approved testing modality with both tissue- and liquid-based options to identify common targetable genetic alterations. Plasma-based liquid biopsies are advantageous as patients can be easily followed over the course of management; resistant clones and related mutations can be identified early, leading to therapy change.[28] Foundation Liquid and Guardant360 commercial assays can detect MSI-high disease and actionable alterations in DNA repair enzymes relevant to clinical decision-making in men with progressive mCRPC and are recommended when tissue testing is unavailable/insufficient.[82,83]

Although the potential for biomarkers or measures of lineage plasticity and NEPC transformation or tumor genotyping is evident, further clinical trials are necessary to appropriately incorporate our developing understanding into clinical practice. Numerous AR-targeted approaches are presently under study, including ARV-110, an AR-degrading PROTAC therapy (NCT05177042 and NCT03888612), CBP/p300 inhibitors that block AR signaling (NCT03568656), bispecific antibodies targeting AR-dependent cell surface antigens such as PSMA or STEAP1 (ie, NCT05125016, NCT04221542, etc.), PSMA-directed CAR-T cells (NCT04429451, etc.) or Lu177 radioligand therapies (NCT03454750, etc.), and many more.[84] As we better comprehend the mechanisms of both primary and acquired resistance in CRPC, both decision-making and treatments used in this disease will continue to be optimized.

SUMMARY

Advanced PCa is complex with a variety of molecular mechanisms associated with CRPC therapeutic resistance. Certain mechanisms are primary in nature, whereas others are acquired, driven by selective pressures of the current treatments. Resistance has been shown in both AR-mediated and non-AR-mediated fashions. Ongoing and future efforts will be critical to gain a deeper understanding and inform clinical practice.

CLINICS CARE POINTS

- Despite newer androgen receptor (AR)-targeted therapies for metastatic castrate-resistant prostate cancer (mCRPC), many patients do not experience treatment response and most eventually experience secondary resistance

- Various AR-related and AR-unrelated mechanisms of resistance in CRPC have been identified
- Further study is needed to identify clinically actionable biomarkers, ideal combinations of treatments to circumvent resistance patterns, and other novel therapeutic agents

DISCLOSURE

Dr A.J. Armstrong has the following disclosures: Research support (to Duke) from the NIH/NCI, PCF/Movember, DOD, Astellas, Pfizer, Bayer, Janssen, Dendreon, Genentech/Roche, BMS, AstraZeneca, Merck, Constellation, BeiGene, Forma, Celgene, Amgen. Consulting or advising relationships with Astellas, Epic Sciences, Pfizer, Bayer, Janssen, Dendreon, BMS, AstraZeneca, Merck, Forma, Celgene, Clovis, and Exact Sciences. The other authors have no disclosures. All authors have read and approved the manuscript, which is not under consideration elsewhere. No specific funding was allocated to this work.

REFERENCES

1. Nakazawa M, Paller C, Kyprianou N. Mechanisms of Therapeutic Resistance in Prostate Cancer. Curr Oncol Rep 2017;19(2):13.
2. Vellky JE, Ricke WA. Development and prevalence of castration-resistant prostate cancer subtypes. Neoplasia 2020;22(11):566–75.
3. Scher HI, Beer TM, Higano CS, et al. Antitumour activity of MDV3100 in castration-resistant prostate cancer: a phase 1-2 study. Lancet 2010;375(9724):1437–46.
4. Efstathiou E, Titus M, Wen S, et al. Molecular characterization of enzalutamide-treated bone metastatic castration-resistant prostate cancer. Eur Urol 2015;67(1):53–60.
5. Buttigliero C, Tucci M, Bertaglia V, et al. Understanding and overcoming the mechanisms of primary and acquired resistance to abiraterone and enzalutamide in castration resistant prostate cancer. Cancer Treat Rev 2015;41(10):884–92.
6. Zhang T, Zhu J, George DJ, et al. Enzalutamide versus abiraterone acetate for the treatment of men with metastatic castration-resistant prostate cancer. Expert Opin Pharmacother 2015;16(4):473–85.
7. Antonarakis ES, Lu C, Wang H, et al. AR-V7 and resistance to enzalutamide and abiraterone in prostate cancer. N Engl J Med 2014;371(11):1028–38.
8. Bluemn EG, Coleman IM, Lucas JM, et al. Androgen Receptor Pathway-Independent Prostate Cancer Is Sustained through FGF Signaling. Cancer Cell 2017;32(4):474–89.e6.
9. Aggarwal R, Huang J, Alumkal JJ, et al. Clinical and Genomic Characterization of Treatment-Emergent Small-Cell Neuroendocrine Prostate Cancer: A Multi-institutional Prospective Study. J Clin Oncol 2018;36(24):2492–503.
10. Csizmarik A, Hadaschik B, Kramer G, et al. Mechanisms and markers of resistance to androgen signaling inhibitors in patients with metastatic castration-resistant prostate cancer. Urol Oncol 2021;39(10):728 e13–e24.
11. Nakazawa M, Antonarakis ES, Luo J. Androgen receptor splice variants in the era of enzalutamide and abiraterone. Horm Cancer 2014;5(5):265–73.
12. Li Y, Yang R, Henzler CM, et al. Diverse AR Gene Rearrangements Mediate Resistance to Androgen Receptor Inhibitors in Metastatic Prostate Cancer. Clin Cancer Res 2020;26(8):1965–76.
13. Dehm SM, Schmidt LJ, Heemers HV, et al. Splicing of a novel androgen receptor exon generates a constitutively active androgen receptor that mediates prostate cancer therapy resistance. Cancer Res 2008;68(13):5469–77.
14. Kim EH, Cao D, Mahajan NP, et al. ACK1-AR and AR-HOXB13 signaling axes: epigenetic regulation of lethal prostate cancers. NAR Cancer 2020;2(3):zcaa018.
15. Scher HI, Graf RP, Schreiber NA, et al. Assessment of the Validity of Nuclear-Localized Androgen Receptor Splice Variant 7 in Circulating Tumor Cells as a Predictive Biomarker for Castration-Resistant Prostate Cancer. JAMA Oncol 2018;4(9):1179–86.
16. Armstrong AJ, Halabi S, Luo J, et al. Prospective Multicenter Validation of Androgen Receptor Splice Variant 7 and Hormone Therapy Resistance in High-Risk Castration-Resistant Prostate Cancer: The PROPHECY Study. J Clin Oncol 2019;37(13):1120–9.
17. Antonarakis ES, Lu C, Luber B, et al. Androgen Receptor Splice Variant 7 and Efficacy of Taxane Chemotherapy in Patients With Metastatic Castration-Resistant Prostate Cancer. JAMA Oncol 2015;1(5):582–91.
18. Armstrong AJ, Luo J, Nanus DM, et al. Prospective Multicenter Study of Circulating Tumor Cell AR-V7 and Taxane Versus Hormonal Treatment Outcomes in Metastatic Castration-Resistant Prostate Cancer. JCO Precis Oncol 2020;4. PO.20.00200.
19. Azad AA, Volik SV, Wyatt AW, et al. Androgen Receptor Gene Aberrations in Circulating Cell-Free DNA: Biomarkers of Therapeutic Resistance in Castration-Resistant Prostate Cancer. Clin Cancer Res 2015;21(10):2315–24.
20. Waltering KK, Urbanucci A, Visakorpi T. Androgen receptor (AR) aberrations in castration-resistant

prostate cancer. Mol Cell Endocrinol 2012;360(1–2): 38–43.

21. Jayaram A, Wingate A, Wetterskog D, et al. Plasma Androgen Receptor Copy Number Status at Emergence of Metastatic Castration-Resistant Prostate Cancer: A Pooled Multicohort Analysis. JCO Precis Oncol 2019;3. PO.19.00123.

22. Kohli M, Li J, Du M, et al. Prognostic association of plasma cell-free DNA-based androgen receptor amplification and circulating tumor cells in pre-chemotherapy metastatic castration-resistant prostate cancer patients. Prostate Cancer Prostatic Dis 2018;21(3):411–8.

23. Takeda DY, Spisak S, Seo JH, et al. A Somatically Acquired Enhancer of the Androgen Receptor Is a Noncoding Driver in Advanced Prostate Cancer. Cell 2018;174(2):422–432 e13.

24. Dang HX, Chauhan PS, Ellis H, et al. Cell-free DNA alterations in the AR enhancer and locus predict resistance to AR-directed therapy in patients with metastatic prostate cancer. JCO Precis Oncol 2020;4:680–713.

25. Galletti G, Leach BI, Lam L, et al. Mechanisms of resistance to systemic therapy in metastatic castration-resistant prostate cancer. Cancer Treat Rev 2017;57:16–27.

26. Bohl CE, Wu Z, Miller DD, et al. Crystal structure of the T877A human androgen receptor ligand-binding domain complexed to cyproterone acetate provides insight for ligand-induced conformational changes and structure-based drug design. J Biol Chem 2007;282(18):13648–55.

27. Korpal M, Korn JM, Gao X, et al. An F876L mutation in androgen receptor confers genetic and phenotypic resistance to MDV3100 (enzalutamide). Cancer Discov 2013;3(9):1030–43.

28. Carreira S, Romanel A, Goodall J, et al. Tumor clone dynamics in lethal prostate cancer. Sci Transl Med 2014;6(254):254ra125.

29. Cai C, Chen S, Ng P, et al. Intratumoral de novo steroid synthesis activates androgen receptor in castration-resistant prostate cancer and is upregulated by treatment with CYP17A1 inhibitors. Cancer Res 2011;71(20):6503–13.

30. Chen EJ, Sowalsky AG, Gao S, et al. Abiraterone treatment in castration-resistant prostate cancer selects for progesterone responsive mutant androgen receptors. Clin Cancer Res 2015;21(6):1273–80.

31. Farla P, Hersmus R, Trapman J, et al. Antiandrogens prevent stable DNA-binding of the androgen receptor. J Cell Sci 2005;118(Pt 18):4187–98.

32. Chen L, Mooso BA, Jathal MK, et al. Dual EGFR/HER2 inhibition sensitizes prostate cancer cells to androgen withdrawal by suppressing ErbB3. Clin Cancer Res 2011;17(19):6218–28.

33. Zhang Z, Karthaus WR, Lee YS, et al. Tumor Microenvironment-Derived NRG1 Promotes Antiandrogen Resistance in Prostate Cancer. Cancer Cell 2020;38(2):279–296 e9.

34. Nikhil K, Haymour HS, Kamra M, et al. Phosphorylation-dependent regulation of SPOP by LIMK2 promotes castration-resistant prostate cancer. Br J Cancer 2021;124(5):995–1008.

35. Stopsack KH, Nandakumar S, Wibmer AG, et al. Oncogenic Genomic Alterations, Clinical Phenotypes, and Outcomes in Metastatic Castration-Sensitive Prostate Cancer. Clin Cancer Res 2020;26(13):3230–8.

36. Wen S, Niu Y, Huang H. Posttranslational regulation of androgen dependent and independent androgen receptor activities in prostate cancer. Asian J Urol 2020;7(3):203–18.

37. Karantanos T, Evans CP, Tombal B, et al. Understanding the mechanisms of androgen deprivation resistance in prostate cancer at the molecular level. Eur Urol 2015;67(3):470–9.

38. Araujo JC, Trudel GC, Saad F, et al. Docetaxel and dasatinib or placebo in men with metastatic castration-resistant prostate cancer (READY): a randomised, double-blind phase 3 trial. Lancet Oncol 2013;14(13):1307–16.

39. Ueda T, Mawji NR, Bruchovsky N, et al. Ligand-independent activation of the androgen receptor by interleukin-6 and the role of steroid receptor coactivator-1 in prostate cancer cells. J Biol Chem 2002;277(41):38087–94.

40. Fizazi K, De Bono JS, Flechon A, et al. Randomised phase II study of siltuximab (CNTO 328), an anti-IL-6 monoclonal antibody, in combination with mitoxantrone/prednisone versus mitoxantrone/prednisone alone in metastatic castration-resistant prostate cancer. Eur J Cancer 2012;48(1):85–93.

41. Gui B, Gui F, Takai T, et al. Selective targeting of PARP-2 inhibits androgen receptor signaling and prostate cancer growth through disruption of FOXA1 function. Proc Natl Acad Sci U S A 2019; 116(29):14573–82.

42. Pan W, Zhang Z, Kimball H, et al. Abiraterone Acetate Induces CREB1 Phosphorylation and Enhances the Function of the CBP-p300 Complex, Leading to Resistance in Prostate Cancer Cells. Clin Cancer Res 2021;27(7):2087–99.

43. Welti J, Sharp A, Brooks N, et al. Targeting the p300/CBP Axis in Lethal Prostate Cancer. Cancer Discov 2021;11(5):1118–37.

44. Pernigoni N, Zagato E, Calcinotto A, et al. Commensal bacteria promote endocrine resistance in prostate cancer through androgen biosynthesis. Science 2021;374(6564):216–24.

45. Logothetis CJ, Gallick GE, Maity SN, et al. Molecular classification of prostate cancer progression: foundation for marker-driven treatment of prostate cancer. Cancer Discov 2013;3(8):849–61.

46. Thomas L, Sharifi N. Germline HSD3B1 Genetics and Prostate Cancer Outcomes. Urology 2020;145:13–21.

47. Mostaghel EA, Marck BT, Plymate SR, et al. Resistance to CYP17A1 inhibition with abiraterone in castration-resistant prostate cancer: induction of steroidogenesis and androgen receptor splice variants. Clin Cancer Res 2011;17(18):5913–25.

48. Chang KH, Li R, Papari-Zareei M, et al. Dihydrotestosterone synthesis bypasses testosterone to drive castration-resistant prostate cancer. Proc Natl Acad Sci U S A 2011;108(33):13728–33.

49. Stanbrough M, Bubley GJ, Ross K, et al. Increased expression of genes converting adrenal androgens to testosterone in androgen-independent prostate cancer. Cancer Res 2006;66(5):2815–25.

50. Jin R, Yamashita H, Yu X, et al. Inhibition of NF-kappa B signaling restores responsiveness of castrate-resistant prostate cancer cells to anti-androgen treatment by decreasing androgen receptor-variant expression. Oncogene 2015; 34(28):3700–10.

51. Carver BS, Chapinski C, Wongvipat J, et al. Reciprocal feedback regulation of PI3K and androgen receptor signaling in PTEN-deficient prostate cancer. Cancer Cell 2011;19(5):575–86.

52. Sweeney C, Bracarda S, Sternberg CN, et al. Ipatasertib plus abiraterone and prednisolone in metastatic castration-resistant prostate cancer (IPATential150): a multicentre, randomised, double-blind, phase 3 trial. Lancet 2021;398(10295): 131–42.

53. Di Mitri D, Mirenda M, Vasilevska J, et al. Re-education of Tumor-Associated Macrophages by CXCR2 Blockade Drives Senescence and Tumor Inhibition in Advanced Prostate Cancer. Cell Rep 2019;28(8): 2156–21568 e5.

54. Li Y, He Y, Butler W, et al. Targeting cellular heterogeneity with CXCR2 blockade for the treatment of therapy-resistant prostate cancer. Sci Transl Med 2019;11(521). eaax0428.

55. Valle S, Sharifi N. Targeting Glucocorticoid Metabolism in Prostate Cancer. Endocrinology 2021; 162(9). bqab132.

56. Serritella AV, Shevrin D, Heath EI, et al. Phase I/II trial of enzalutamide and mifepristone, a glucocorticoid receptor antagonist, for metastatic castration-resistant prostate cancer. Clin Cancer Res 2022; 28(8):1549–59.

57. Mu P, Zhang Z, Benelli M, et al. SOX2 promotes lineage plasticity and antiandrogen resistance in TP53- and RB1-deficient prostate cancer. Science 2017; 355(6320):84–8.

58. Beltran H, Prandi D, Mosquera JM, et al. Divergent clonal evolution of castration-resistant neuroendocrine prostate cancer. Nat Med 2016;22(3):298–305.

59. Davies A, Nouruzi S, Ganguli D, et al. An androgen receptor switch underlies lineage infidelity in treatment-resistant prostate cancer. Nat Cell Biol 2021;23(9):1023–34.

60. Ku SY, Rosario S, Wang Y, et al. Rb1 and Trp53 cooperate to suppress prostate cancer lineage plasticity, metastasis, and antiandrogen resistance. Science 2017;355(6320):78–83.

61. Komiya A, Yasuda K, Watanabe A, et al. The prognostic significance of loss of the androgen receptor and neuroendocrine differentiation in prostate biopsy specimens among castration-resistant prostate cancer patients. Mol Clin Oncol 2013;1(2): 257–62.

62. Abida W, Cyrta J, Heller G, et al. Genomic correlates of clinical outcome in advanced prostate cancer. Proc Natl Acad Sci U S A 2019;116(23): 11428–36.

63. Adams EJ, Karthaus WR, Hoover E, et al. FOXA1 mutations alter pioneering activity, differentiation and prostate cancer phenotypes. Nature 2019; 571(7765):408–12.

64. Brown LC, Halabi S, Schonhoft JD, et al. Circulating Tumor Cell Chromosomal Instability and Neuroendocrine Phenotype by Immunomorphology and Poor Outcomes in Men with mCRPC Treated with Abiraterone or Enzalutamide. Clin Cancer Res 2021; 27(14):4077–88.

65. Brennen WN, Zhu Y, Coleman IM, et al. Resistance to androgen receptor signaling inhibition does not necessitate development of neuroendocrine prostate cancer. JCI Insight 2021;6(8). e146827.

66. Beltran H, Oromendia C, Danila DC, et al. A Phase II Trial of the Aurora Kinase A Inhibitor Alisertib for Patients with Castration-resistant and Neuroendocrine Prostate Cancer: Efficacy and Biomarkers. Clin Cancer Res 2019;25(1):43–51.

67. Puca L, Gavyert K, Sailer V, et al. Delta-like protein 3 expression and therapeutic targeting in neuroendocrine prostate cancer. Sci Transl Med 2019;11(484). eaav0891.

68. Robinson D, Van Allen EM, Wu YM, et al. Integrative clinical genomics of advanced prostate cancer. Cell 2015;161(5):1215–28.

69. Cheng HH, Pritchard CC, Boyd T, et al. Biallelic Inactivation of BRCA2 in Platinum-sensitive Metastatic Castration-resistant Prostate Cancer. Eur Urol 2016;69(6):992–5.

70. de Bono J, Mateo J, Fizazi K, et al. Olaparib for Metastatic Castration-Resistant Prostate Cancer. N Engl J Med 2020;382(22):2091–102.

71. Chakraborty G, Armenia J, Mazzu YZ, et al. Significance of BRCA2 and RB1 Co-loss in Aggressive Prostate Cancer Progression. Clin Cancer Res 2020;26(8):2047–64.

72. Saad F, Armstrong AJ, Thiery-Vuillemin A, et al. PROpel: Phase III trial of olaparib (ola) and abiraterone (abi) versus placebo (pbo) and abi as first-line (1L) therapy for patients (pts) with metastatic castration-resistant prostate cancer (mCRPC). J Clin Oncol 2022;40(6_suppl):11.

73. Chi KN, Rathkopf DE, Smith MR, et al. Phase 3 MAGNITUDE study: First results of niraparib (NIRA) with abiraterone acetate and prednisone (AAP) as first-line therapy in patients (pts) with metastatic castration-resistant prostate cancer (mCRPC) with and without homologous recombination repair (HRR) gene alterations. J Clin Oncol 2022;40(6_suppl):12.

74. Pritchard CC, Morrissey C, Kumar A, et al. Complex MSH2 and MSH6 mutations in hypermutated microsatellite unstable advanced prostate cancer. Nat Commun 2014;5:4988.

75. Graff JN, Alumkal JJ, Drake CG, et al. Early evidence of anti-PD-1 activity in enzalutamide-resistant prostate cancer. Oncotarget 2016;7(33): 52810–7.

76. Abida W, Cheng ML, Armenia J, et al. Analysis of the Prevalence of Microsatellite Instability in Prostate Cancer and Response to Immune Checkpoint Blockade. JAMA Oncol 2019;5(4):471–8.

77. Chen WS, Aggarwal R, Zhang L, et al. Genomic Drivers of Poor Prognosis and Enzalutamide Resistance in Metastatic Castration-resistant Prostate Cancer. Eur Urol 2019;76(5):562–71.

78. Miyamoto DT, Zheng Y, Wittner BS, et al. RNA-Seq of single prostate CTCs implicates noncanonical Wnt signaling in antiandrogen resistance. Science 2015;349(6254):1351–6.

79. Paller C, Pu H, Begemann DE, et al. TGF-beta receptor I inhibitor enhances response to enzalutamide in a pre-clinical model of advanced prostate cancer. Prostate 2019;79(1):31–43.

80. Gundem G, Van Loo P, Kremeyer B, et al. The evolutionary history of lethal metastatic prostate cancer. Nature 2015;520(7547):353–7.

81. Drake JM, Graham NA, Lee JK, et al. Metastatic castration-resistant prostate cancer reveals intrapatient similarity and interpatient heterogeneity of therapeutic kinase targets. Proc Natl Acad Sci U S A 2013;110(49):E4762–9.

82. Sonpavde G, Agarwal N, Pond GR, et al. Circulating tumor DNA alterations in patients with metastatic castration-resistant prostate cancer. Cancer 2019; 125(9):1459–69.

83. Ritch E, Fu SYF, Herberts C, et al. Identification of Hypermutation and Defective Mismatch Repair in ctDNA from Metastatic Prostate Cancer. Clin Cancer Res 2020;26(5):1114–25.

84. Labriola MK, Atiq S, Hirshman N, et al. Management of men with metastatic castration-resistant prostate cancer following potent androgen receptor inhibition: a review of novel investigational therapies. Prostate Cancer Prostatic Dis 2021;24(2):301–9.

Testosterone and Male Sexual Function

Logan B. Galansky, MD[a],*, Jason A. Levy, DO, MS[b], Arthur L. Burnett, MD, MBA[c,d]

KEYWORDS

- Testosterone • Male sexual function • Erectile dysfunction • Ejaculatory dysfunction • Low libido

KEY POINTS

- Testosterone is the driving hormone of male sexual development and function. It has functions in the central nervous system, peripheral nervous system, and end organs.
- The male sexual response cycle is complex and the exact role of testosterone in mediating libido, arousal, erection, ejaculation, and orgasm is multifactorial.
- For men presenting with sexual dysfunction, it is important for clinicians to understand the signs and symptoms and appropriate work-up for low testosterone.

INTRODUCTION

Male sexual function involves a complex interplay between hormonal, anatomic, and neuropsychologic functions and mediators. At the basis of any discussion surrounding normal and abnormal male sexual function is the "male sexual hormone," testosterone (T). Hypogonadism, defined broadly as testicular failure with androgen deficiency, can disrupt the male sexual response cycle as well as normal systemic physiology. The resulting signs and symptoms can include decreased libido, erectile dysfunction, ejaculatory dysfunction, infertility, fatigue, decreased bone density, decreased lean body mass, increased body fat, and sleep disturbances.[1]

The most widely accepted model of the human sexual response cycle was developed by Masters and Johnson in 1996. They described a four-stage linear process through the phases of arousal, plateau, orgasm, and resolution.[1] Some frameworks, such as that proposed by Singer Kaplan, also include a desire phase which precedes the arousal phase.[2]

For men, the corresponding physiologic processes to the sexual response cycle are libido and sexual desire, arousal and erection, and ejaculation and orgasm. These physiologic functions are mediated by central and peripheral nervous system pathways, end-organ motor and sensory mechanisms, and molecular signaling pathways of the vascular system.

Basics of Testosterone

T is the main bioavailable androgen circulating in men. Most of the circulating T is produced by Leydig cells in the testis, with a smaller amount synthesized by the adrenal glands.[3] Testicular synthesis of T is dependent on a functional hypothalamic–pituitary–gonadal (HPG) axis. Beginning in the hypothalamus, gonadotropin-releasing hormone (GnRH) is secreted, stimulating the production of luteinizing hormone (LH) in the gonadotropic basophil cells of the anterior pituitary gland.[4] LH then acts on the Leydig cells in the testis to stimulate the production of T. T, and its metabolite estradiol (E2), then act to inhibit

a Johns Hopkins School of Medicine Brady Urological Institute, The Johns Hopkins Hospital, 600 North Wolfe Street, Baltimore, MD 21287, USA; b Johns Hopkins School of Medicine Brady Urological Institute, The Johns Hopkins Hospital, 600 North Wolfe Street Park 2, Baltimore, MD 21287, USA; c Oncology Center, Johns Hopkins School of Medicine Brady Urological Institute, The Johns Hopkins Hospital, 600 North Wolfe Street, Marburg 407, Baltimore, MD 21287, USA; d Johns Hopkins Clinical Research Network, 1830 Monument Street, Suite 328, Baltimore, MD 21205, USA
* Corresponding author.
E-mail address: lgalans1@jhmi.edu
Twitter: @LoganGalanskyMD (L.B.G.)

Urol Clin N Am 49 (2022) 627–635
https://doi.org/10.1016/j.ucl.2022.07.006
0094-0143/22/Published by Elsevier Inc.

GnRH and LH secretion at the hypothalamus and pituitary gland as well as downstream T secretion by Leydig cells in a standard negative feedback loop.[4]

Once produced by the Leydig cells, T can circulate freely, become bound to carrier molecules, or undergo conversion to its main metabolites, dihydrotestosterone (DHT) and E2. T is converted to DHT by the enzyme 5-alpha reductase and to estradiol by the enzyme aromatase in various tissues throughout the body, including the prostate, liver, skin, testis, adipose tissue, and brain, respectively. It is then that T, DHT, and E2 can act directly on target tissues, primarily by binding to the androgen receptor. Free T accounts for 1–2% of circulating T that is unbound. Of the remaining circulating T, approximately 60% is bound to sex hormone binding globulin (SHBG), with the remaining bound to albumin and other serum proteins. Only circulating T that is free or albumin-bound is biochemically available to act on target tissues.[5]

T and its metabolites act throughout the body on multiple organ systems, including muscle, bone, skin, brain, and peripheral nerves. It is also essential for the development of the male phenotype, male puberty, male sexual function, and spermatogenesis.

Role of Testosterone in Male Sexual Anatomy Development

Male sexual anatomy development is influenced by T as early as the eighth week in utero.[5] During this time, Leydig cells differentiate from genital ridge cells and begin to produce T. Serum and testicular T levels continue to rise between the 8th and 13th week to maintain the Wolffian duct system and stimulate the development of the male external genitalia, male accessory sexual tissues (seminal vesicles, prostate, bulbourethral glands), male reproductive tract tissues (testes, epididymides, vas deferens, ejaculatory ducts), and pelvic floor structures (pelvic diaphragm muscles). After 13 weeks gestation, T levels begin to decline.[5]

Studies have shown that T regulates the differentiation of penile stem cells to the smooth muscle phenotype that is necessary to form the functional and structural anatomy for penile erection.[6] In developmental and adult rodent castration models, penile architecture is compromised as demonstrated by lower intracorporal peak pressures following cavernous nerve stimulation compared with noncastrate animals.[7]

In prepubertal men, T levels remain low at less than 30 ng/dL.[8] During adolescence, puberty and further development of male secondary sex characteristics are triggered by pulsatile hypothalamic GnRH, with respondent increases in T levels to 100–300 ng/dL during puberty and levels greater than 300 ng/dL as an adult.[9]

The sympathetic and parasympathetic nerves that supply the urogenital organs form the major pelvic ganglia. These autonomic nerves arise from the spinal preganglionic neurons of the lumbar and sacral spinal cord and control erection, ejaculation, and detumescence.[9] During late gestation and in the early postnatal period, T contributes to proper pelvic ganglia formation, and thereby sexual reflexes.[8,10]

MALE SEXUAL FUNCTION PHYSIOLOGY: ROLE OF TESTOSTERONE
Physiologic Mechanisms

Despite numerous studies investigating the physiology of the male sexual response cycle, the exact role of T in mediating the steps of the process remains incompletely known. However, the literature suggests that T is key in coordinating the processing of sexual libido, the mechanics of erections, and ejaculatory function.

The first stage of the sexual response cycle involves sexual desire and libido. Sexual desire is influenced by many factors, including psychosocial, cultural, and situational, whereas libido is a biologic response directly related to T levels. Mediation of libido by T occurs in the central nervous system. Studies have shown expression of the androgen receptor in key brain areas, including the amygdala, preoptic area, and paraventricular nucleus of the hypothalamus.[10]

It has also been demonstrated that T is involved in the physiology of erections, most likely through its influence on molecular mediators of erectile function, formation of penile architecture, and activity of smooth muscle pathways.[8] T has been shown to influence enzymatic activity in the corpora cavernosa that is responsible for both erection and detumescence.[8] In hypogonadal animal models, T regulates the formation of molecules involved with erection, namely nitric oxide (NO), RhoA-ROCK, and PDE5.[8] Castration models have also demonstrated the downregulation of the NO/cyclic guanosine monophosphate(cGMP) pathway in conjunction with other T-dependent biologic effects, causing smooth muscle and endothelial apoptosis and lipofibrosis of the penile corpora cavernosa that results in corporal veno-occlusive dysfunction.[11]

The neural networks involved in ejaculation include both peripheral pelvic and genital nerves as well as galaninergic neurons in the central spinal cord.[12] It has been suggested that the formation of galaninergic neurons is at least partially androgen-mediated, as studies of female and male cadavers show a greater density of galaninergic neurons in the L3–L4 segments of male spinal cords.[13] Lesions to these structures have been associated with ejaculatory failure despite penile stimulation.[13] The ejaculatory reflex is coordinated by neuromuscular mediators in the hypothalamic nuclei, specifically serotoninergic and dopaminergic neurons, responsible for inhibition and promotion, respectively.[14] In the peripheral nervous system, emission and expulsion are then controlled by sympathetic and parasympathetic pathways.[15] In rat models and some human studies examining ejaculatory dysfunction, T deficiency has been associated with decreased dopaminergic response, leading to a delay in orgasmic function, as dopaminergic neurons facilitate the central ejaculatory reflex.[13] It has been hypothesized that low T is associated with increased inhibitory tone in male genital smooth muscle cells, which subsequently contributes to delayed ejaculation.[16]

MALE SEXUAL DYSFUNCTION PATHOPHYSIOLOGY: ROLE OF TESTOSTERONE
Libido Dysfunction (Symptomatic Hypogonadism)

Libido plays a critical role in initiating the male sexual response cycle. Low libido is characterized by a persistent deficient desire for sexual activity. This can be experienced in isolation, as with hypoactive sexual desire disorder, or as one symptom among a cluster of problems, as in symptomatic hypogonadism. Prevalence of low libido in men is variable with studies reporting between 5 and 17% of men endorsing problems with libido and other aspects of sexual desire, and further diminishing libido with increasing age.[15]

The American Urologic Association (AUA) defines T deficiency as < 300 ng/dL.[17] In men with T deficiency, diminished libido is a common sexual symptom. Although the exact mechanism of T's effect on libido remains unknown, studies have shown that in men undergoing androgen deprivation therapy (ADT), libido is severely impacted with only 5% of men maintaining a high level of sexual interest.[18] Moreover, many human and animal castration studies have demonstrated the connection between hypogonadism and decreased libido.[8] A study on T and hypogonadism found that as T drops below a threshold of 15 nmol/L (433 ng/dL), men can start experiencing loss of libido. Interestingly, libido seems to be one of the early signs of hypogonadism as other symptoms, such as changes in sleep, concentration and mood, obesity and diabetes, and erectile dysfunction, are not observed until T levels drop below 8–12 nmol/L (231–346 ng/dL).[19] Thus, T has been linked to sexual behaviors and connecting these behaviors when an appropriate stimulus is present. As such, in men diagnosed with hypogonadism, treatment with T supplementation has been shown to improve libido along with other sexual symptoms.[17] Interestingly, in eugonadal men with low libido, over-supplementation with exogenous T was not shown to improve sexual drive, suggesting that there are multiple factors underlying male hypoactive sexual desire.[17]

Erectile Dysfunction

Erectile dysfunction (ED) is defined as, "an impairment in the arousal phase of [the male] sexual response" with "consistent or recurrent inability to attain and/or maintain penile erection sufficient for sexual satisfaction, including satisfactory sexual performance."[20]

The prevalence of ED has been widely reported by a variety of sources. Approximately 20 percent of adult men are reported to have ED.[21]

ED is typically classified as psychogenic or organic.[22] The pathogenesis of ED is multifactorial and can involve multiple underlying disturbances, including vasculogenic, neurogenic, hormonal, and/or medication-induced.

Although most men with ED do not have hypogonadism, ED has been shown to be related to low T levels in some cases. It has been postulated that T may exert local effects to mediate erections based on studies demonstrating fluctuations in serum and corporal T levels during erection.[23] Studies have shown that once T drops below a threshold of roughly 230 ng/dL, men can begin to experience ED.[21] This is particularly relevant for men undergoing ADT, for whom ED is a well-established potential side effect. Further research is being undertaken to better understand the mechanisms by which hypogonadism affects erectile function.

Ejaculatory Dysfunction

Disorders of ejaculation arise when a man does not have control of ejaculation and if there is distress by the man or sexual partner related to ejaculation.[24] Based on when and if ejaculation occurs it can be classified as retrograde ejaculation, premature ejaculation, delayed ejaculation, or failure of ejaculation/anejaculation.

The AUA and Sexual Medicine Society of North America (SMSNA) 2020 guideline on disorders of ejaculation primarily details premature and delayed ejaculation. It defines premature ejaculation (PE) as, "poor ejaculatory control, associated bother, and ejaculation within about 2 minutes of the initiation of penetrative sex that has been present since sexual debut."[24]

The epidemiology of PE has been challenging to capture due to the confounding factors of perceived PE and normal ejaculation latency time. Thus, although 30% of men have self-reported PE, most men have ejaculation latency times greater than two minutes.[25] In turn, the actual prevalence of PE for those having distress is likely around 5%, but this does not discount that men with PE experience substantial distress.[25] The exact pathophysiology of PE is not known. However, similar to ED, the hypothesized risk factors can be psychologic, neurologic, hormonal, and medication-related.

The understanding of the effect of T on ejaculatory response is limited, but some studies have shown that higher T levels are correlated with premature ejaculation while lower levels are associated with delayed ejaculation in humans.[26] A randomized controlled trial of testosterone replacement therapy (TRT) in hypogonadal men found improvements in ejaculatory function, although perceived bother remained unchanged.[27] Additionally, there is evidence to suggest that T may act on peripheral and central pathways that impact ejaculatory response time by increasing arousal, regulating CNS effects, and changing seminal fluid volume.[8]

In contrast to PE, some men may experience delayed ejaculation (DE), defined as, "lifelong, consistent, bothersome inability to achieve ejaculation, or excessive latency of ejaculation, despite adequate sexual stimulation and desire to ejaculate."[25]

The epidemiology of DE is similarly difficult to capture as DE often exists concurrently with low libido or ED and is therefore underreported. According to the Global Survey of Sexual Attitudes and Beliefs, approximately 14% of men aged 40–80 years old reported difficulty attaining orgasm.[25]

The pathophysiology of DE can be related to problems with sexual stimulation resulting in complications with emission and expulsion. Risk factors that contribute to DE are increasing age, medications, drugs, or neurologic suppression of the normal CNS arousal responses that produce sexual climax, ED, lower urinary tract symptoms, hypothyroidism, and low serum T. In one systematic review, low T levels were significantly associated with mild to moderate DE and a history of hypogonadism doubled a man's relative risk for DE.[28]

CLINICAL EVALUATION OF LOW TESTOSTERONE

Men presenting with issues related to sexual function should undergo a comprehensive evaluation, including medical, surgical, and social history, medication reconciliation, physical examination, and laboratory/adjunct studies as indicated.

History

A focused patient history should be the first step in evaluation. Assessing for T deficiency should include questions related to both sexual and nonsexual symptoms. As described above, low libido, ED, and problems with ejaculation are often commonly attributed to low T. Other symptoms, such as decreased energy, irritability or depression, and weight gain may also be signs of T deficiency.

Validated questionnaires can be useful in further elucidating sexual history. For example, the International Index of Erectile Function (IIEF), Sexual Health Inventory for Men (SHIM), and Erection Hardness Score (EHS) are frequently used in the assessment of ED. Importantly, when discussing a patient's sexual history, it is imperative to understand any psychological or interpersonal factors that may be contributing to the patient's symptoms before any additional work-up.

There are questionnaires focusing on screening for low T in general, though they should not be used to determine if patients are candidates for TRT per AUA guidelines. Common hypogonadism questionnaires include the androgen deficiency in the aging male (ADAM) questionnaire, the Aging Male's Symptoms (AMS) scale, and the New England Research Institute (NERI) Hypogonadism Screener.[29] Notably, while these screening tools have relatively strong sensitivity, ranging from 59 to 97%, the specificity differs widely from 19 to 59%, resulting in varying degrees of success in predicting hypogonadism.[30] Consequently, a quantitatively-proven low T level continues to be the first line for diagnosing hypogonadism.[30]

Social history should involve discussion of any recreational drug or alcohol use, current or prior use of anabolic steroids, and any occupational exposures as certain substances can influence T levels.

Surgical history should focus on both procedures involving the pelvis and testicles (e.g., prostatectomy, orchiectomy, pelvic radiation, and so forth) as well as the brain (e.g., intracranial surgery or radiation, pituitary surgery). It is also useful to discuss the relevant history of any trauma to the testicles or genitals, as this can affect sexual function.

A general overview of the patient's other chronic health conditions, or common signs of undiagnosed conditions associated with sexual dysfunction (e.g. claudication for peripheral vascular disease), should be undertaken.

Reviewing the patient's current medication list is important as certain medications can affect sexual function and T synthesis, particularly corticosteroids, selective serotonin reuptake inhibitors, opioids, chemotherapeutics, and aldosterone receptor antagonists, among others (**Box 1**).

Physical Examination

As with any physical exam, vital signs should be evaluated. Deviations in secondary male sexual characteristics, such as lack of facial and pubic hair, decreased muscle distribution, and gynecomastia, can suggest possible T deficiency. If there is a concern for ED, palpation of peripheral pulses, abdominal exam for abdominal aortic aneurysm, and neurologic exam for neuropathy should be performed as ED can be a harbinger of cardiovascular or neurologic disease.

Although a physical exam can be normal in men with T deficiency, a comprehensive genital exam should be performed. The penis should be thoroughly examined with careful palpation of the shaft to evaluate for any deformities or plaques consistent with Peyronie's disease. The penis should also be examined for any skin lesions or urethral meatus abnormalities. The scrotal exam should include the assessment of testicular size, consistency, and location, as well as the evaluation for the presence of any testicular masses or other abnormalities, such as varicocele. In men reporting lower urinary tract symptoms or who are being considered for possible TRT, a digital rectal exam to evaluate the prostate for any abnormalities can be performed.

Box 1
Medications associated with hypogonadism

Corticosteroids (e.g., dexamethasone)

Psychotropic medications (e.g., paroxetine, amitriptyline)

Opioids (e.g., oxycodone)

Alkylating agents (e.g., cisplatin)

Aldosterone receptor antagonists (e.g., spironolactone)

H_2-receptor antagonists (e.g., cimetidine)

Antifungals (e.g., ketoconazole)

Substance use (e.g., marijuana, nicotine, anabolic steroids)

Laboratory Tests

Current AUA guidelines recommend obtaining 2 morning serum total T levels on separate occasions as the initial screening for T deficiency.[15] If the total T level is < 300 ng/dL and the patient is experiencing signs and/or symptoms of low T, this is consistent with a diagnosis of T deficiency.[15] Moreover, in men presenting with ED, total T concentration can be useful in detecting underlying hypogonadism and informing treatment options.

There is some debate regarding testing for free T levels in the setting of normal total T concentrations. As total T concentrations can be affected by SHBG levels, some experts advocate for measuring free T when clinical suspicion for T deficiency is high, despite normal total T levels. Free T can be measured directly by radioimmunoassay (RIA), liquid chromatography, equilibrium dialysis, or calculated indirectly using total T and SHBG concentrations. There can be significant variability in free T reference ranges, but in general, RIA free T levels < 1.0–1.5 ng/dL and calculated free T levels < 80–100 pg/mL are consistent with T deficiency in symptomatic men.[31] It is important to note that current AUA guidelines do not recommend treatment for T deficiency based on low free T levels alone and clinical judgment should be used based on symptoms and patient-specific risks and benefits of trialing TRT.

In evaluating for T deficiency, additional tests can be considered to help differentiate between primary, secondary, and compensated T deficiency. These can include LH, prolactin, FSH, estradiol, thyroid function studies (TSH, T3, T4), and hematocrit.[32] In men over the age of 40 years old who may be started on TRT, prostate-specific antigen (PSA) screening should be considered to establish a baseline.[33] In men desiring fertility, semen analysis can also be considered before starting TRT to determine semen quality, as exogenous T use can suppress spermatogenesis.[34]

As noted above, T deficiency can have deleterious effects on many organ systems and ED can be a preceding symptom of other undiagnosed medical comorbidities. As a result, it is reasonable for clinicians to also obtain a complete blood count, basic metabolic panel, serum glucose, hemoglobin A1c, and lipid panel. While any derangements in these studies may not change the treatment options for T deficiency or ED, they can help identify related medical conditions that may require attention.

Similarly, in asymptomatic men presenting with unexplained medical conditions, such as anemia, bone density loss, HIV/AIDS, male infertility, or diabetes, or who have known risk factors for T deficiency, such as history of chemotherapy, pelvic/testicular radiation, chronic opioid use, or chronic steroid use, it may be prudent to obtain labs to investigate for T deficiency.

Other Studies

For patients with T deficiency, additional testing is based on laboratory and exam findings. For instance, pituitary MRI should be obtained if low T levels are found concurrently with abnormal prolactin, FSH, or LH levels. Karyotype studies can be considered if men have small firm testes and other phenotypic changes suggestive of Klinefelter syndrome on examination. For patients presenting with ED, adjunct neurologic or vascular testing may be warranted.

TREATMENT OPTIONS FOR MALE SEXUAL DYSFUNCTION

Interest in TRT has increased dramatically over the past decade and has been a topic of much debate among the FDA, general practitioners, and the urologic community. In general, the AUA/SMSNA guidelines state that TRT can be safely used for adult-onset hypogonadism with careful monitoring of treatment efficacy and side effects.[33]

Low Libido

Meta-analyses investigating the effect of TRT on male sexual function have demonstrated variable improvements in libido. In these studies, TRT led to reported improvements specifically in hypogonadal men, with no change in libido for eugonadal men.[32] Furthermore, the benefits of TRT were found to be greater in men with lower baseline levels of T (< 288 ng/dL).[35] Although the literature suggests that TRT can improve libido in hypogonadal men, some studies have shown no significant difference in sexual satisfaction after TRT.[36]

Erectile Dysfunction

In hypogonadal men, TRT has been shown to improve responses to PDE5 inhibitors (PDE5i) for ED.[37] Several randomized controlled trials and systematic reviews of hypogonadal men with ED have shown that PDE5i therapy in conjunction with TRT is more effective in improving ED than PDE5i therapy or TRT alone.[24,28] Therefore, the AUA recommends that urologists inform hypogonadal men with ED that PDE5i therapy may be augmented by TRT.[24]

While TRT in hypogonadal men may optimize the efficacy of other ED treatments by restoring normal T levels, there is not adequate data to support combining TRT with other ED treatments.

Similarly, TRT is not recommended as a monotherapy for ED.[30]

Ejaculatory Disorders

Some studies have shown the benefits of TRT on ejaculatory function in hypogonadal men.[38] AUA/SMSNA guidelines on ejaculatory disorders state that clinicians can offer TRT in men with DE and T deficiency.[39]

It is important to note that there is no evidence-based target T level for hypogonadal men with DE, but a T level at or above the 50th percentile (>500–550 ng/dL) is recommended unless symptoms improve at lower T levels. If TRT is to help with DE symptoms, clinical improvements are typically observed within 90 days of achieving eugonadal T levels. TRT is not indicated in eugonadal men with DE per AUA/SMSNA guidelines.[40]

CONSIDERATIONS FOR SPECIAL POPULATIONS

While the clinical evaluation will be largely the same for any man presenting with sexual dysfunction, it is prudent to consider several specific circumstances that may alter the clinician's approach to evaluating concerns of low T.

Men with Medical Chronic Health Conditions

Adult-onset hypogonadism (AOH) occurs more frequently in men who have a history of chronic disease.[41] In particular, metabolic syndrome, obesity, and renal failure are some of the most common conditions associated with AOH.[3,41]

Metabolic syndrome is a collection of risk factors for heart disease, stroke, and type 2 diabetes, defined as high blood pressure, increased fasting glucose, central obesity, and dyslipidemia.[42] In the United States, the incidence of metabolic syndrome has steadily increased with over 34% of adults diagnosed with the disorder and a 38% incidence of obesity among American men.[43] Metabolic syndrome can cause secondary hypogonadism for a variety of reasons. For obese men, in particular, aromatization of T in adipose cells leads to higher physiologic levels of estrogen and resultant low libido, ED, and ejaculatory dysfunction in these men.[41]

Renal failure has a similar effect on the hypothalamic–pituitary–gonadal axis. While hypogonadism in renal failure is again multifactorial, it has been demonstrated that renal failure causes decreased production of LH and decreased prolactin clearance, both of which hinder T production.[44] Studies have shown that hypogonadism is associated with increased morbidity and mortality in men with renal failure, due to systemic effects of low T such as anemia, reduced bone density and muscle mass, and premature cardiovascular disease.[35] Although the risk–benefit ratio is controversial, in appropriately selected patients with renal failure, TRT has been shown to help normalize hormonal parameters, decrease medical morbidity, and improve sexual dysfunction.[45]

Men After Radical Prostatectomy

Pelvic surgery, and specifically radical prostatectomy, can impact erectile function, ejaculatory function, and orgasmic function to varying degrees depending on the patient's preoperative baseline as well as the surgical approach.

In treating men who present with low T after radical prostatectomy, it is important to understand the theoretical risk of TRT on prostate cancer recurrence. Presently, both the AUA and European Association of Urology (EAU) have posited that the current literature does not demonstrate clear evidence connecting T to the development of prostate cancer.[17,40] That being said, current practice guidelines recommend considering TRT postprostatectomy only in those men with favorable pathology (ie. negative margins, negative seminal vesicle involvement, negative lymph nodes) who have undetectable postoperative PSA levels.[15] This is based on a series of studies demonstrating that in patients started on TRT who had undergone radical prostatectomy with undetectable postoperative PSA levels, there was no rise in PSA or recurrence of prostate cancer.[36,46,47] For men on active surveillance, the literature suggests that TRT is not associated with the progression of prostate cancer in men with low volume and low-to-moderate grade cancer when used for a limited amount of time.[48] TRT may be harmful in men with advanced diseases who are on active surveillance protocols.[49]

Overall, it is essential that the clinician engages in shared-decision making with the patient the risks and benefits of TRT when treating symptomatic hypogonadal men with a history of prostate cancer.

Transgender Patients

Transgender patients pose unique work-up and treatment considerations as the hormonal milieu has been medically and/or surgically altered depending on the patient's stage of transition.

For transgender men (female-to-male transition), the goal of gender affirmation hormonal therapy is to increase serum T levels to a male-appropriate range and suppress estrogen levels. This is accomplished with both medical TRT (target physiologic T level of 300–1000 ng/dL) and surgical estrogen suppression (ie. bilateral oophorectomy). TRT can be delivered parenterally or transdermally, using testosterone cypionate, testosterone undecanoate, or testosterone gel or patch, with regular laboratory monitoring.[50]

As with cisgender men undergoing TRT, transgender men experience phenotypic and neuropsychiatric changes. In regards to sexual function, TRT most notably can cause increased libido and irreversible clitoral hypertrophy (in patients who have not yet undergone masculinizing genital gender affirmation surgery). Erectile function is dependent on the creation of a neophallus and implantation of an implantable penile prosthesis.

For transgender women (male-to-female transition), hormonal therapy involves androgen deprivation and estrogen supplementation. Androgen deprivation is achieved medically with GnRH analogs, spironolactone, or cyproterone acetate and surgically with bilateral orchiectomy.[43] Estrogen is typically administered transdermally to minimize the cardiovascular risks associated with oral estrogen therapy.

It is important to note that removal of the prostate and seminal vesicles is not a standard procedure in feminizing genital gender affirmation surgery. As a result, transgender women can still be at risk for prostate cancer. For urologists taking care of these patients, the World Professional Association for Transgender Health (WPATH) recommends using current prostate cancer screening guidelines for cisgender men regarding age and risk stratification when counseling transgender women.[51] Importantly, WPATH recommends that the PSA upper threshold of normal in transgender women should be set at 1 ng/mL.[46] This recommendation was established based on evidence that a biopsy positive for prostate cancer despite a low PSA value is more common in the setting of T deficiency, which is akin to the hormonal status of transgender women.[46] Finally, WPATH advises transvaginal prostate palpation over DRE in patients who have undergone gender affirmation surgery given the altered anatomy.[46]

CLINICS CARE POINTS

- Work-up for men with sexual dysfunction should include a thorough history and physical examination, with particular focus on signs and symptoms of low T, common medical comorbidities, and physical exam findings suggestive of hormonal imbalance.

- Low T can present with sexual and nonsexual symptoms. In patients presenting with signs and symptoms of low T, clinicians should obtain two-morning serum total T levels, with values < 300 ng/dL indicative of low T.

- AUA/SMSNA guidelines state that TRT may improve low libido, ED (when paired with PDE5i therapy), and DE in hypogonadal men, but is not recommended in eugonadal men.

- Certain special patient populations, including men with metabolic syndrome, men who have undergone radical prostatectomy, and transgender patients may require additional assessment and testing.

- Our understanding of the complex role of T in the male sexual response cycle and the pathophysiology of sexual dysfunction is evolving and can help inform clinicians on current and future treatments for patients.

DISCLOSURE

The authors have nothing to disclose.

REFERENCES

1. Masters WH, Johnson VE. Human sexual response. Boston: Little, Brown; 1966.
2. Kaplan HS. The new sex therapy: active treatment of sexual dysfunctions. London: Routledge; 1974.
3. Alex Tatem MD. Testosterone deficiency: physiology, epidemiology, pathophysiology, and evaluation - Sexual Medicine and andrology: Urology core curriculum. Available at: https://university.auanet.org/core/sexual-medicine-andrology/testosterone-deficiency-physiology-epidemiology-pathophysiology-and-evaluation/index.cfm. Accessed January 24, 2022.
4. Matsumoto AM, Bremner WJ. Testicular disorders. In: Melmed S, Polansky KS, Larsen PR, et al, editors. Williams textbook of endocrinology. New York: Elsevier; 2016. p. 688–777.
5. Ceccarelli F. The embryology of the genitalia. AUA Update Ser 1982;1(26):2–6.
6. Corona G, Maggi M. The role of testosterone in erectile dysfunction. Nature News. 2009. Available at: https://www.nature.com/articles/nrurol.2009.235. Accessed January 24, 2022.
7. Podlasek CA, Mulhall J, Burnett AL, et al. Translational perspective on the role of testosterone in sexual function and dysfunction. J Sex Med 2016. Available at: https://www.ncbi.nlm.nih.gov/pmc/articles/PMC5333763/. Accessed January 24, 2022.
8. Bhasin S, Cunningham GR, Hayes FJ, et al. Testosterone therapy in adult men with androgen deficiency syndromes: an endocrine society clinical practice guideline. J Clin Endocrinol Metab 2010; 95(6):2356–9.
9. Keast JR. Plasticity of pelvic autonomic ganglia and urogenital innervation. Int Rev Cytol 2006;248: 141–208.
10. Swaab DF. Sexual differentiation of the brain and behavior. Best Pract Res Clin Endocrinol Metab 2007;21:431–44.
11. Kovanecz I, Ferrini MG, Vernet D, et al. Pioglitazone prevents corporal veno-occlusive dysfunction in a rat model of type 2 diabetes mellitus. BJU Int 2006;98:116–24.
12. Chehensse C, Facchinetti P, Bahrami S, et al. Human spinal ejaculation generator. Ann Neurol 2017; 81:35.
13. Sato Y, Shibuya A, Adachi H, et al. Restoration of sexual behavior and dopaminergic neurotransmission by long term exogenous testosterone replacement in aged male rats. J Urol 1998;160: 1572–5.
14. Ralph DJ, Wylie KR. Ejaculatory disorders and sexual function. BJU Int 2005;95(9):1181–6.
15. Hypoactive sexual desire disorder. Mestonlabcom. Available at: https://labs.la.utexas.edu/mestonlab/hypoactive-sexual-desire-disorder/#:~:text=Prevalence%20rates%20typically%20decrease%20when,%2C%20%26%20Moreira%2C%202009)). Accessed January 24, 2022.
16. Corona G. Psychobiological correlates of delayed ejaculation in male patients with sexual dysfunctions. J Androl 2006;27(3):453–8.
17. Testosterone deficiency guideline - american urological association. Available at: https://www.auanet.org/guidelines/guidelines/testosterone-deficiency-guideline. Accessed January 24, 2022.
18. Potosky A, Knopf K, Clegg L, et al. Quality of life outcomes after primary androgen deprivation therapy: results from the prostate cancer outcomes study. J Clin Oncol 2001;19:3750–7.
19. Zitzmann M, Faber S, Nieschlag E. Association of specific symptoms and metabolic risks with serum testosterone in older men. J Clin Endocrinol Metab 2006;91(11):4335–43.
20. Erectile dysfunction (ED) guideline - american urological association. Available at: https://www.auanet.org/guidelines/guidelines/erectile-dysfunction-(ed)-guideline. Accessed January 24, 2022.
21. Selvin E, Burnett AL, Platz EA. Prevalence and risk factors for erectile dysfunction in the US. Am J Med 2007;120(2):151–7.
22. MacDonald SM, Burnett AL. Physiology of erection and pathophysiology of erectile dysfunction. Surg Clin North Am 2021;48(4):513–25.
23. Becker AJ, Ückert S, Stief CG, et al. Cavernous and systemic testosterone levels in different phases of human penile erection. Urology 2000;56(1):125–9.

24. Guideline statements. Disorders of ejaculation: an AUA/SMSNA guideline - american urological association. Available at: https://www.auanet.org/guidelines/guidelines/disorders-of-ejaculation. Accessed January 24, 2022.

25. Nicolosi A, Buvat J, Glasser DB, et al. Sexual behaviour, sexual dysfunctions and related help seeking patterns in middle-aged and elderly Europeans: the global study of sexual attitudes and behaviors. World J Urol 2006;24:423.

26. Corona G, Jannini EA, Lotti F, et al. Premature and delayed ejaculation: two ends of a single continuum influenced by hormonal milieu. Int J Androl 2010;34: 41–8.

27. Maggi M, Heiselman D, Knorr J, et al. Impact of testosterone solution 2% on ejaculatory dysfunction in hypogonadal men. J Sex Med 2016;13(8): 1220–6. https://doi.org/10.1016/j.jsxm.2016.05.012.

28. Spitzer M, Basaria S, Travison TG, et al. Effect of testosterone replacement on response to sildenafil citrate in men with erectile dysfunction. Ann Intern Med 2012;157(10):681.

29. Sterling J, Bernie AM, Ramasamy R. Hypogonadism: easy to define, hard to diagnose, and controversial to treat, 2015 treat. Can Urol Assoc J 2015; 9(1–2):65–8.

30. Boloña ER, Uraga MV, Haddad RM, et al. Testosterone use in men with sexual dysfunction: a systematic review and meta-analysis of randomized placebo-controlled trials. Mayo Clin Proc 2007; 82(1):20–8.

31. Morgentaler A. Commentary: guideline for male testosterone therapy: a clinician's perspective. J Clin Endocrinol Metab 2007;92:416–7.

32. Isidori AM, Giannetta E, Gianfrilli D, et al. Effects of testosterone on sexual function in men: results of a meta-analysis. Clin Endocrinol 2005;63(4):381–94.

33. Khera M, Broderick GA, Carson CC, et al. Adult-onset hypogonadism. Mayo Clin Proc 2016;91(7): 908–26.

34. Tatem AJ, Beilan J, Kovac JR, et al. Management of anabolic steroid-induced infertility: novel strategies for Fertility Maintenance and recovery. World J Men's Health 2020;38(2):141.

35. Snyder PJ, Bhasin S, Cunningham GR, et al. Effects of testosterone treatment in older men. N Engl J Med 2016;374(7):611–24.

36. Agarwal PK, Oefelein MG. Testosterone replacement therapy after primary treatment for prostate cancer. J Urol 2005;173:533.

37. Buvat J, Montorsi F, Maggi M, et al. Hypogonadal men nonresponders to the PDE5 inhibitor Tadalafil benefit from normalization of testosterone levels with a 1% hydroalcoholic testosterone gel in the treatment of erectile dysfunction (TADTEST study). J Sex Med 2011;8(1):284–93.

38. Corona G, Isidori AM, Buvat J, et al. Testosterone supplementation and sexual function: a meta-analysis study. J Sex Med 2014;11:1577–92.

39. Disorders of ejaculation guideline – american urological association. Available at: https://www.auanet.org/guidelines/guidelines/disorders-of-ejaculation. Accessed January 24, 2022.

40. Salonia A, Bettocchi C, Boeri L, et al. European association of urology guidelines on sexual and reproductive health—2021 update: Male sexual dysfunction. Eur Urol 2021;80(3):333–57.

41. Freedland SJ, Aronson WJ. Examining the relationship between obesity and prostate cancer. Rev Urol 2004;6(2):73–81.

42. Alberti KGMM, Eckel RH, Grundy SM, et al. Harmonizing the metabolic syndrome. Circulation 2009; 120(16):1640–5.

43. Metabolic syndrome prevalence by race/ethnicity and sex in the United States, National Health and Nutrition Examination Survey, 1988–2012. Centers Dis Control Prev 2017. Available at: https://www.cdc.gov/pcd/issues/2017/16_0287.htm. Accessed January 24, 2022.

44. Snyder G, Shoskes DA. Hypogonadism and testosterone replacement therapy in end-stage renal disease (ESRD) and transplant patients. Transl Androl Urol 2016;5(6):885–9.

45. Thirumavalavan N, Wilken NA, Ramasamy R. Hypogonadism and renal failure: an update. Indian J Urol 2015;31(2):89–93.

46. Kaufman JM, Graydon RJ. Androgen replacement after curative radical prostatectomy for prostate cancer in hypogonadal men. J Urol 2004;172:920.

47. Khera M, Grober ED, Najari B, et al. Testosterone replacement therapy following radical prostatectomy. J Sex Med 2009;6:1165.

48. Morgentaler A, Lipshultz LI, Bennett R, et al. Testosterone therapy in men with untreated prostate cancer. J Urol 2011;185:1256.

49. Kim M, Byun SS, Hong SK. Testosterone replacement therapy in men with untreated or treated prostate cancer: do we have enough evidences? World J Mens Health 2021;39(4):705–23.

50. UCSF Transgender Care, D.o.F.a.C.M., University of California San Francisco. Guidelines for the Primary and Gender-Affirming Care of Transgender and Gender Nonbinary People; 2nd edition. Deutsch MB, ed. June 2016, transcare.ucsf.edu/guidelines.

51. Standards of care - WPATH world professional association. Available at: https://www.wpath.org/media/cms/Documents/SOC%20v7/Standards%20of%20Care%20V7%20-%202011%20WPATH.pdf?_t=1605186324. Accessed January 24, 2022.

What We Have Learned from The Testosterone Trials

Peter J. Snyder, MD

KEYWORDS

- Testosterone • Late-onset hypogonadism • Sexual function • Volumetric bone mineral density
- Hemoglobin

KEY POINTS

- As men age, the serum concentrations of total testosterone decrease only slightly.
- As men age, the serum concentration of sex hormone binding globulin increases, so that the serum concentration of free testosterone decreases more than the total.
- Testosterone treatment of men with late-onset hypogonadism increases all aspects of sexual function, volumetric bone mineral density, and hemoglobin.
- Testosterone treatment only slightly improves walking, vitality, and mood in men with late-onset hypogonadism.
- Testosterone treatment of men with late-onset hypogonadism increases noncalcified coronary artery plaque volume.

TESTOSTERONE DECREASES WITH INCREASING AGE

As men age, their serum testosterone concentrations decrease. Unlike the decrease in estradiol in women at menopause, which is relatively rapid in onset, severe in degree, and the result of primary gonadal failure, the decrease in testosterone in men is gradual, to a modest degree, and the result of combined primary and secondary gonadal failures. Several terms have been applied to this fall in testosterone for no reason other than increasing age, most commonly late-onset hypogonadism.

Serum Total Testosterone

Cross-sectional studies show only a very small decrease in the concentrations of total testosterone with increasing age. The mean serum testosterone concentration fell only 0.04% per year in the European Male Aging Study of men aged 40 to 79 years (**Fig. 1**).[1] A study that combined samples from four other studies of 9054 men aged 19–99 years found that the median serum testosterone concentration decreased only from 507 ng/dL in men 19–39 years old to 446 ng/dL in men 80–99 years old, but the 5th percentile decreased from 273 to 203 ng/dL, and the 2.5th percentile decreased from 229 to 119 ng/dL.[2]

Longitudinal studies show a somewhat greater decrease. In the Baltimore Longitudinal Study on Aging, 890 men experienced a decrease from approximately 519 ng/dL at age 30 to 346 ng/dL at age 80.[3] In the Massachusetts Male Aging Study, men were evaluated over approximately 15 years and were found to have an average decrease in total testosterone concentration of 14.5% per decade.[4]

Although serum testosterone levels do decrease with age, the prevalence of men over age 65 who can be considered to be hypogonadal due to age alone is relatively small.

Division of Endocrinology, Diabetes and Metabolism, Perelman School of Medicine, University of Pennsylvania, 3400 Civic Center Boulevard, Philadelphia, PA 19104, USA
E-mail address: pjs@pennmedicine.upenn.edu

Urol Clin N Am 49 (2022) 637–644
https://doi.org/10.1016/j.ucl.2022.07.007
0094-0143/22/© 2022 Elsevier Inc. All rights reserved.

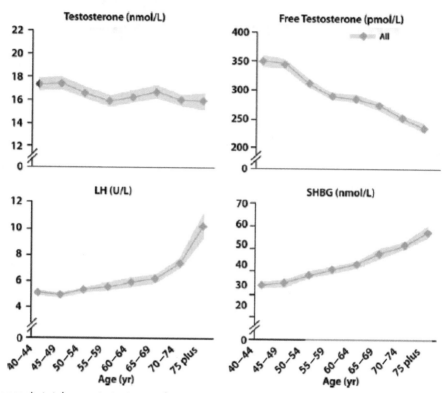

Fig. 1. Changes in total serum testosterone, free serum testosterone, sex hormone binding globulin, and luteinizing hormone serum concentrations as men age in men enrolled in the European Male Aging Study.[1]

Serum Free Testosterone and Sex Hormone Binding Globulin

As men age, their serum concentrations of sex hormone binding globulin (SHBG) gradually increase. In the European Male Aging Study, the increase was about 50% from the early 40s to the late 70s (see **Fig. 1**).[1] Because SHBG binds testosterone with high affinity, free testosterone decreases with age much more than total testosterone (see **Fig. 1**); free testosterone concentrations in men aged 75–79 were approximately 30% lower than those in men aged 40–44.[1]

Serum Luteinizing Hormone

As seen in the European Male Aging Study, serum concentrations of luteinizing hormone remain relatively stable through age 70 but then increase in later years (see **Fig. 1**).[1] The magnitude of the increase, however, is not as great as one would expect from the decrease in free testosterone, suggesting that the decrease in free testosterone is the result of both primary and secondary hypogonadism.

Early Studies of Testosterone Treatment for Late-Onset Hypogonadism

The studies that demonstrated a decrease in serum testosterone levels with increasing age

and the realization that many of the manifestations of old age, such as decreases in sexual function, energy, and osteoporosis, are similar to the consequences of classical hypogonadism, led to trials to determine if testosterone treatment of men with late-onset hypogonadism would convey any benefits. These trials were generally small and showed mixed results. For example, one trial showed that testosterone increased bone mineral density,[5] but two others did not.[6,7] One trial showed that testosterone increased muscle strength, but another did not.[8] In 2003, a committee of the National Academy of Medicine reviewed the data in the field and concluded that the evidence at that time did not show a benefit of testosterone treatment of late-onset hypogonadism.[9] The committee recommended that the National Institutes of Health fund a coordinated set of trials to determine if testosterone treatment of late-onset hypogonadism had any benefit. The committee recommended deferring studies of the possible risks of this treatment unless and until a benefit could be demonstrated.

THE TESTOSTERONE TRIALS

The Testosterone Trials were a set of seven coordinated trials designed to implement the recommendation of the National Academy of Medicine to determine if testosterone treatment of late-onset hypogonadism would have any benefit. The trials were conducted at 12 US clinical trial sites.

Screening for The Testosterone Trials

In this regard, 51,085 men 65 years and older were screened by telephone to find 788 men who eventually met all entry criteria and enrolled.[10] There were many entry criteria, but not having a serum testosterone concentration <275 ng/dL on two morning specimens was the major reason for exclusion; only 14.7% of those who volunteered met this criterion. This low percentage of men who could be considered to have late-onset hypogonadism is consistent with the population studies cited earlier.[2,11] Other reasons for exclusion were moderately severe lower urinary tract symptoms and a relatively high risk of prostate cancer.

Testosterone Treatment

Men who enrolled in The Testosterone Trials were allocated to receive either a testosterone or placebo gel in a double-blind fashion for 1 year.[10] The initial dose of testosterone was 5 g a day. The dose was adjusted to maintain the serum testosterone concentration within the normal range for young men. To maintain the blinding, when a man taking testosterone gel was instructed

to change the dose, a man taking placebo gel was also instructed to change the dose.

In men allocated to take testosterone, the median serum testosterone concentration increased from distinctly, though only moderately, low (231 ng/dL) to the middle of the normal range by month 3 of the trial and remained normal until the end of the trial at 12 months (500–550 ng/dL) (Fig. 2).[10,12] The median serum concentrations of free testosterone and estradiol also increased to mid-normal, and the median concentration of dihydrotestosterone increased to the upper end of the normal range. In men allocated to take placebos, the median concentrations of the hormones did not change.

Parameters that Testosterone Improved Moderately

Testosterone treatment for 1 year improved sexual function, bone density, and hemoglobin.

Sexual function
Testosterone treatment, compared to placebo, significantly increased sexual activity (Fig. 3), libido, and erectile function (erectile dysfunction).[10,12] The increase in sexual activity included all aspects, from flirting to intercourse,[13] and was to a moderate degree, as illustrated by an effect size of 0.43. Increases in sexual activity and libido were significantly associated with increases in

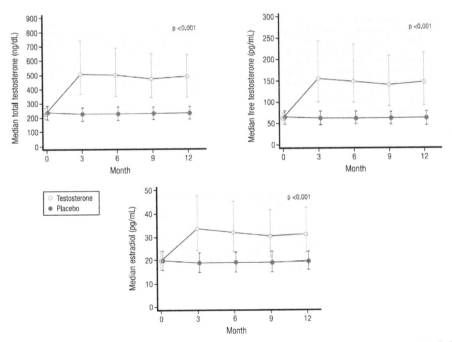

Fig. 2. Serum concentrations of serum total testosterone, serum free testosterone, and serum estradiol during 1 year of treatment with testosterone or placebo in men participating in The Testosterone Trials.[12]

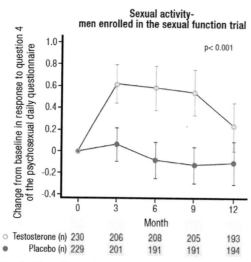

Fig. 3. The effect of testosterone compared to placebo treatment for 1 year on sexual activity in men enrolled in The Testosterone Trials.[12]

total and free testosterone and estradiol. In another trial of testosterone in men whose baseline serum testosterone concentration was 202 ng/dL and had low sexual drive, testosterone treatment of 311 men for 12 weeks increased sexual interest significantly more than placebo treatment of 308 men.[14]

Bone density

Testosterone dramatically improved bone parameters as assessed by quantitative computed tomography.[12,15] The effect was greatest on volumetric bone mineral density, which increased by 6.8% over placebo, and estimated strength of trabecular bone of the lumbar spine, which increased by 8.5% over placebo, both in the lumbar spine (**Fig. 4**). Testosterone also increased volumetric bone mineral density and estimated strength of peripheral bone, which is largely cortical bone, but not quite as much as trabecular bone, and increased these parameters in the hip, but to a lesser degree. During the 1 year of treatment and the subsequent year of observation, the number of fractures in men treated with testosterone was the same as in men treated with placebo, but the number of men and the observation period were too small to draw conclusions about the possible efficacy of testosterone in reducing fractures.

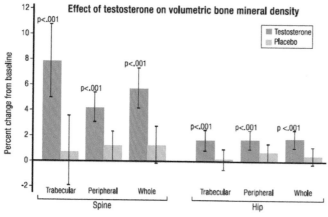

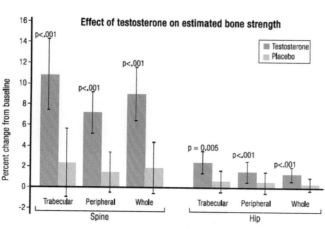

Fig. 4. The effect of testosterone or placebo treatment for 1 year on volumetric bone mineral density (top panel) or estimated bone strength (bottom panel), as determined by quantitative computed tomography in men enrolled in the bone trial of The Testosterone Trials.[12]

Hemoglobin

Testosterone increased hemoglobin by approximately 1 g/dL in men who were anemic at baseline for no discernible reason, but it also increased hemoglobin by the same degree in men who were anemic and had a recognizable cause, such as iron deficiency (**Fig. 5**).[12,16] These results are consistent with the well-established stimulatory effect of testosterone on erythropoiesis. The likely explanation for the increase in hemoglobin in men who had known causes of anemia is that these men, like all men in The Testosterone Trials, also had low serum testosterone concentrations.

Parameters that Testosterone Improved Marginally

Testosterone treatment improved walking, vitality, and mood, but marginally.[10]

Walking

Testosterone treatment compared to placebo did not significantly increase the distance walked in 6 minutes by more than 50 m in men whose walking speed was slow at baseline, but did so in all men. Testosterone also increased the distance walked in 6 minutes in both slow-walking men and all men. Testosterone increased men's perception of their walking ability and their perception of their overall physical functioning, as assessed by the physical function domain of the SF-36 questionnaire. The magnitude of these increases, however, was small, as indicated by effect sizes of 0.08–0.15.

Vitality

Testosterone did not significantly increase the number of men whose scores on the Facit-Fatigue Scale increased by more than 4 points, but it marginally increased the absolute score and increased the vitality score on the SF-36 questionnaire. The magnitude of these effects was small, as indicated by effect sizes of 0.15–0.19.

Mood

Mood was assessed by the positive and negative affect scales. Testosterone increased positive mood but decreased negative mood. Testosterone also decreased depressive symptoms, as measured by the Patient Health Questionnaire 9. All of the increases were to a small degree though.

Parameters that Testosterone Did Not Improve

Cognitive function

In the 493 men in the Testosterone Trials who had age-related memory impairment, testosterone did not improve delayed paragraph recall, immediate paragraph recall, visual memory, spatial ability,

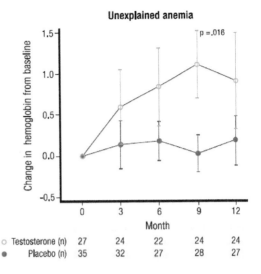

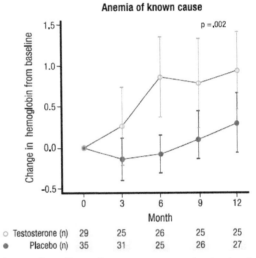

Fig. 5. The effect of testosterone or placebo treatment for 1 year on hemoglobin in men enrolled in The Testosterone Trials who had unexplained anemia or anemia of known cause.[12]

executive function, or subjective memory complaints.[17] In all of the men in the trial, testosterone marginally improved executive function but did not improve any of the other parameters.

Lipids and metabolic parameters

Testosterone treatment had small and inconsistent effects on lipids and metabolic parameters.[18] Testosterone slightly decreased low-density lipoprotein cholesterol but also slightly decreased high-density lipoprotein cholesterol. Testosterone slightly decreased fasting insulin concentration and the homeostatic model assessment of insulin resistance but did not affect fasting glucose or hemoglobin A1c.

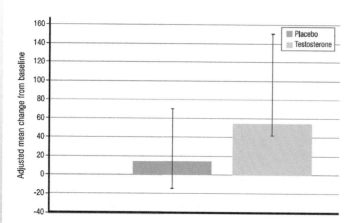

Fig. 6. The effect of testosterone or placebo treatment for 1 year on change in noncalcified coronary artery plaque volume, as determined by computed tomographic angiography in men enrolled in the cardiovascular trial of The Testosterone Trials.[12]

The One Parameter that Testosterone Worsened

Coronary artery plaque volume

Coronary artery plaque volume was assessed by computed tomographic angiography in 138 men in the Testosterone Trials.[19] Testosterone significantly increased noncalcified and total coronary artery plaque volume (**Fig. 6**).[12,19] In The Testosterone Trials overall, the number of major adverse cardiovascular events was the same, in each treatment group, seven, but the number of participants (788) and the 1-year duration of treatment were not sufficient to draw conclusions regarding the cardiovascular safety of testosterone treatment.

The results of other studies are also inconclusive. In two retrospective cohort studies, slightly more men who received testosterone had major adverse cardiovascular events than men who did not,[20,21] but in another retrospective cohort study, there was no increased risk of testosterone use.[22] One clinical trial of testosterone in men with mild mobility limitations was stopped early because more men who were being treated with testosterone sustained cardiovascular events than men treated with placebo,[23] but another trial in a similar population reported few cardiovascular events.[24]

Lessons from The Testosterone Trials

The Testosterone Trials show clearly that testosterone treatment of elderly men who have a distinctly and reproducibly low serum testosterone concentration for no reason other than age has clear efficacy. This treatment improves sexual desire and activity to a moderate degree and increases volumetric bone density and hemoglobin dramatically. There are also small improvements in walking, mood, and depressive symptoms. The risks of testosterone treatment on cardiovascular outcomes, benign prostatic hyperplasia, and prostate cancer, however, are still unknown

and will not be known until studies are conducted on larger numbers of men for longer durations.

Approach to the Patient with Late-Onset Hypogonadism

The clinician is faced with a dilemma in approaching a man who has unequivocally and reproducibly low serum testosterone concentrations in the early morning but no obvious reason other than old age and who has symptoms suggestive of hypogonadism. The Testosterone Trials show clear evidence of modest benefit from testosterone treatment of such a man, but the potential risks of this treatment are not known, and the Food and Drug Administration specifically does not approve testosterone treatment for late-onset hypogonadism. This author recommends applying a more strict criterion for prescribing testosterone to a man who has no obvious cause; specifically, an early morning serum testosterone concentration that is reproducibly less than 200 ng/dL, in addition to suggestive symptoms. The serum testosterone concentration during treatment should be kept in the lower part of the normal range, and prostate parameters should be monitored.

FUNDING

The Testosterone Trials were supported by grants from the National Institutes of Aging, National Heart, Lung, and Blood Institute, National Institute of Neurologic Diseases and Stroke, and National Institute of Child Health and Human Development AbbVie provided funding and AndroGel and placebo gel.

CLINICS CARE POINT

- Although testosterone treatment of men with late-onset hypogonadism improves sexual function, volumetric bone mineral density, and hemoglobin to a moderate degree and vitality, mood, and walking slightly, the cardiovascular and prostate risks of this treatment are not known. Until those risks are known, this author recommends testosterone treatment of men with late-onset hypogonadism only if the symptoms are severe and the serum testosterone concentration is less than 200 ng/dL.

DISCLOSURE

The author has nothing to disclose.

REFERENCES

1. Wu FC, Tajar A, Pye SR, et al. Hypothalamic-pituitary-testicular axis disruptions in older men are differentially linked to age and modifiable risk factors: the European Male Aging Study. J Clin Endocrinol Metab 2008;93(7):2737–45.
2. Travison TG, Vesper HW, Orwoll E, et al. Harmonized reference ranges for circulating testosterone levels in men of four cohort studies in the united states and europe. J Clin Endocrinol Metab 2017;102(4): 1161–73.
3. Harman SM, Metter EJ, Tobin JD, et al. Baltimore Longitudinal Study of A. Longitudinal effects of aging on serum total and free testosterone levels in healthy men. Baltimore Longitudinal Study of Aging. J Clin Endocrinol Metab 2001;86(2):724–31.
4. Feldman HA, Longcope C, Derby CA, et al. Age trends in the level of serum testosterone and other hormones in middle-aged men: longitudinal results from the Massachusetts male aging study. J Clin Endocrinol Metab 2002;87(2):589–98. Available at: http://www.ncbi.nlm.nih.gov/htbin-post/Entrez/query?db=m&form=6&dopt=r&uid=11836290 http://jcem.endojournals.org/cgi/content/full/87/2/589 http://jcem.endojournals.org/cgi/content/abstract/87/2/589.
5. Amory JK, Watts NB, Easley KA, et al. Exogenous testosterone or testosterone with finasteride increases bone mineral density in older men with low serum testosterone. J Clin Endocrinol Metab 2004; 89(2):503–10. Available at: http://www.ncbi.nlm.nih.gov/entrez/query.fcgi?cmd=Retrieve&db=PubMed&dopt=Citation&list_uids=14764753.
6. Snyder PJ, Peachey H, Hannoush P, et al. Effect of testosterone treatment on bone mineral density in men over 65 years of age. J Clin Endocrinol Metab 1999;84(6):1966–72. Available at: http://www.ncbi.nlm.nih.gov/htbin-post/Entrez/query?db=m&form=6&dopt=r&uid=10372695.
7. Kenny AM, Prestwood KM, Gruman CA, et al. Effects of transdermal testosterone on bone and muscle in older men with low bioavailable testosterone levels. J Gerontol

A Biol Sci Med Sci 2001;56(5):M266–72. Available at: http://www.ncbi.nlm.nih.gov/htbin-post/Entrez/query?db=m&form=6&dopt=r&uid=11320105.
8. Snyder PJ, Peachey H, Hannoush P, et al. Effect of testosterone treatment on body composition and muscle strength in men over 65 years of age. J Clin Endocrinol Metab 1999;84(8):2647–53. Available at: http://www.ncbi.nlm.nih.gov/htbin-post/Entrez/query?db=m&form=6&dopt=r&uid=10443654.
9. Liverman CTBD. Testosterone and aging. Washington, DC: Institute of Medicine of the National Academies; 2003.
10. Snyder PJ, Bhasin S, Cunningham GR, et al. Effects of testosterone treatment in older men. N Engl J Med 2016;374(7):611–24.
11. Wu FC, Tajar A, Beynon JM, et al. Identification of late-onset hypogonadism in middle-aged and elderly men. N Engl J Med 2010;363(2):123–35.
12. Snyder PJ, Bhasin S, Cunningham GR, et al. Lessons from the testosterone trials. Endocr Rev 2018; 39(3):369–86. https://doi.org/10.1210/er.2017-00234.
13. Cunningham GR, Stephens-Shields AJ, Rosen RC, et al. Testosterone Treatment and Sexual Function in Older Men With Low Testosterone Levels. J Clin Endocrinol Metab 2016;101(8): 3096–104.
14. Brock G, Heiselman D, Maggi M, et al. Effect of testosterone solution 2% on testosterone concentration, sex drive and energy in hypogonadal men: results of a placebo controlled study. J Urol 2016; 195(3):699–705.
15. Snyder PJ, Kopperdahl DL, Stephens-Shields AJ, et al. Effect of testosterone treatment on volumetric bone density and strength in older men with low testosterone: a controlled clinical trial. JAMA Intern Med 2017;177(4):471–9. https://doi.org/10.1001/jamainternmed.2016.9539.
16. Roy CN, Snyder PJ, Stephens-Shields AJ, et al. Association of testosterone levels with anemia in older men: a controlled clinical trial. JAMA Intern Med 2017;177(4):480–90.
17. Resnick SM, Matsumoto AM, Stephens-Shields AJ, et al. Testosterone treatment and cognitive function in older men with low testosterone and age-associated memory impairment. JAMA 2017; 317(7):717–27.
18. Mohler ER 3rd, Ellenberg SS, Lewis CE, et al. The effect of testosterone on cardiovascular biomarkers in the testosterone trials. J Clin Endocrinol Metab 2018; 103(2):681–8.
19. Budoff MJ, Ellenberg SS, Lewis CE, et al. Testosterone treatment and coronary artery plaque volume in older men with low testosterone. JAMA 2017; 317(7):708–16.
20. Finkle WD, Greenland S, Ridgeway GK, et al. Increased risk of non-fatal myocardial infarction

following testosterone therapy prescription in men. PLoS One 2014;9(1):e85805.

21. Vigen R, O'Donnell CI, Baron AE, et al. Association of testosterone therapy with mortality, myocardial infarction, and stroke in men with low testosterone levels. JAMA 2013;310(17):1829–36.

22. Shores MM, Smith NL, Forsberg CW, et al. Testosterone treatment and mortality in men with low testosterone levels. J Clin Endocrinol Metab 2012; 97(6):2050–8.

23. Basaria S, Harman SM, Travison TG, et al. Effects of testosterone administration for 3 years on subclinical atherosclerosis progression in older men with low or low-normal testosterone levels: a randomized clinical trial. JAMA 2015; 314(6):570–81.

24. Srinivas-Shankar U, Roberts SA, Connolly MJ, et al. Effects of testosterone on muscle strength, physical function, body composition, and quality of life in intermediate-frail and frail elderly men: a randomized, double-blind, placebo-controlled study. J Clin Endocrinol Metab 2010;95(2): 639–50.

Androgenic Steroids Use and Abuse
Past, Present, and Future

Arthi Thirumalai, MBBS*, Bradley D. Anawalt, MD

KEYWORDS

• Anabolic steroid abuse • Androgens • Doping • Performance-enhancing drugs

KEY POINTS

- Elite athletes commonly abuse androgenic steroids as performance-enhancing drugs and use a variety of tactics to avoid discovery but methods and processes to detect abuse of these performance-enhancing drugs have evolved.
- Among the general population, long-term abuse of androgenic steroids seems to be uncommon but the highest risk groups are teenage boys and young men who are in competitive sports or who are bodybuilders and weightlifters.
- When used at high doses for prolonged periods, there are detrimental effects on the reproductive axis and potentially on the cardiovascular, hepatic, hematologic, neuropsychiatric, and dermatologic systems.
- Androgenic steroid abuse must be distinguished from the use of physiologic dosages for male hypogonadism.
- Androgens at physiologic or near physiologic dosages are generally safe and might also be useful in the chronic catabolic states, sarcopenia, hypoproliferative anemia, and as a component of male hormonal contraceptives.

INTRODUCTION

The effects of androgens have been an area of great interest ever since Charles Edouard Brown reported marked improvements in energy and vigor after self-administering an aqueous extract of canine and bovine testes in the 1870s. In 1935, Ernst Laqueur isolated and Adolf Butenandt and Leopold Ruzicka synthesized testosterone.[1] Subsequently, from the 1950s onwards, athletes started using various chemical derivatives of testosterone for competitive advantage. Although scientists remained skeptical of the effects of these chemicals, athletes continued their widespread use until these drugs were officially banned from use by the International Olympics Committee in 1974.[2] The effects of supraphysiologic testosterone on muscle size and strength were convincingly demonstrated in 1996 by Bhasin and colleagues.[3] It is noteworthy that all androgens have anabolic action at the muscle but the ratio of androgenic to anabolic effects vary by agent (refer to "Muscle-Wasting Conditions" section). Therefore, the term "anabolic androgenic steroids (AASs)" can be condensed to "androgenic steroids,"; however, we have chosen to use "AAS" in this review because readers are likely more familiar with that. AAS abuse spans a wide array of products with the principal goal of increasing systemic androgenic action, by either providing exogenous androgens or their precursors, or by increasing endogenous androgen concentrations (**Fig. 1**). The World Anti-Doping Agency (WADA) was established in 1999 to combat abuse of AASs and performance-enhancing drugs. Despite these measures, androgen abuse remains a

Department of Medicine, University of Washington, 1959 Northeast Pacific Street, HSB C-209, UW Box # 357138, Seattle, WA 98195, USA
* Corresponding author.
E-mail address: arthidoc@uw.edu

Urol Clin N Am 49 (2022) 645–663
https://doi.org/10.1016/j.ucl.2022.07.008
0094-0143/22/© 2022 Elsevier Inc. All rights reserved.

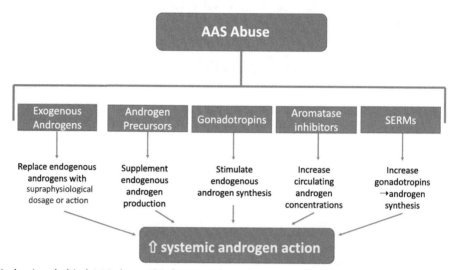

Fig. 1. Mechanisms behind AAS abuse. This figure outlines the various classes of drugs and their mechanisms of increasing systemic androgen effects. AAS, anabolic androgenic steroids; SERMs, selective estrogen receptor modulators.

problem in international sports, and the detection of performance-enhancing chemicals has needed to constantly evolve. Furthermore, the use of AASs has also spilled over into the general population in men aiming to achieve a "desired" appearance and boost self-esteem. There can be adverse consequences of the long-term abuse of AASs. In this review, we will outline the current state of AAS abuse among the general population and in the world of sports, provide guidance on how to diagnose AAS abuse, and offer strategies to manage patients wishing to discontinue their use and attend to their fertility goals during this process. We will also review the consequences of chronic AAS abuse and explore the data behind the therapeutic use of AAS in certain disease states. For this review, we will focus on AAS abuse in men because the prevalence among women is significantly lower[4] and data on long-term consequences and management is of insufficient quality to make strong recommendations.

EPIDEMIOLOGY OF ANABOLIC ANDROGENIC STEROID ABUSE

Estimating the prevalence of AAS use is challenging. Sources of this information include self-reported surveys, results of doping tests, investigative journalism, and government hearings.[5] Limitations of surveys include underreporting due to unwillingness to report,[6,7] small sample sizes, and confusion regarding exact AAS agents used.[8] Using results of doping tests to define the prevalence of AAS use are fraught with issues of variability in lists of banned substances and methodologies of drug testing, and they likely underestimate drug use in elite athletes by 8-fold.[7] Anabolic agents comprise most atypical findings (87%) reported by WADA and all adverse analytical findings (46%) reported by the International Amateur Athletics Foundation per the 2017 Anti-Doping Testing Figures Report.

Among the various studies, prevalence rates of AAS abuse among elite athletes and gym attendees have ranged from 9% to 67% and from 3.5% to 80%, respectively.[9] Weightlifters, powerlifters, and bodybuilders are also at higher risk for chronic AAS abuse, and rates as high as 33% to 80% have been reported.[10,11] Studies looking at these higher risk populations skew the overall prevalence estimates of AAS abuse because these are several-fold higher than in the general population.[4]

It has been estimated that the lifetime prevalence of "ever use" of AAS in the United States is between 1.3 and 4 million with ~100,000 new users annually.[12,13] However, most data do not clearly distinguish among lifetime, one-time, or sporadic use from chronic, sustained use of AAS. A study using mathematical modeling suggests that 30% to 35% of AAS users have used them at doses high enough and durations long enough to cause dependence.[13] The prevalence in the United States might be higher than other parts of the world: lifetime prevalence of AAS use of 0.7% in men and 0.002% in women was reported in a 2012 Swedish national survey of the general population.[14] Men have much higher prevalent use than women in all regions of the world, with a 2014 meta-analysis of worldwide studies of

AAS use indicating a lifetime prevalent use of 6.4% in men and 1.4% in women.[4] However, this study did not distinguish between sporadic use versus chronic abuse of AAS.

Despite the easier access to AAS through the Internet, the overall prevalence of AAS use seems to be declining among adolescents after a peak in the early 2000s.[15] Surveys such as Monitoring the Future and the Youth Risk Behavior Survey showed peaks of 3% to 5% around 2001 and rates around 1% to 3% in 2017 to 2018.[5,16] In summary, although AAS abuse exists in the context of performance-enhancement, there is no epidemic of their use among the general population.

BEHAVIORS AMONG ANABOLIC ANDROGENIC STEROID ABUSERS

AAS abusers tend to have a variety of motivating factors that can include performance-enhancement in athletics and sports, change in bodily appearance with fat-burning and muscle-building or an interest in looking and feeling "better."[17,18] The agents can be procured from multiple sources, with the most commonly reported ones being the Internet (71%), from a gym dealer (24%), foreign mail-order (19%), or prescription (11%).[19,20] Most users overwhelmingly report using (91%–95%) and preferring (77%) injectable options.[19,20] Users often "stack" multiple agents together or "pyramid" by progressively increasing drug intake, plateau, and then taper down during a median cycle length of 11 weeks (average 4–20 weeks) and repeat these patterns for a variable number of cycles (cycling).[5,19,20] The rationale of stacking or pyramiding is based on the incorrect belief that these patterns of use might mitigate against long-term adverse effects. During the "off-cycle" periods, many will consume ancillary drugs: (1) aromatase inhibitors to reduce side effects such as gynecomastia or (2) selective estrogen receptor modulators (SERMs) or gonadotropins (human chorionic gonadotropin [hCG]) to preserve testicular size and enhance testosterone levels, thereby preventing withdrawal symptoms. They may also consume a considerable number of nutraceuticals. An exhaustive list of all these agents and AASs is published elsewhere,[5] and a concise list of commonly abused AASs is presented in **Table 1**. Unfortunately, an overwhelming 92% of AAS users reported that they did not think their physicians were knowledgeable about AAS use.[19] The burden lies with the medical community to bridge this lack of trust, highlight the potential negative effects of prolonged AAS use, identify, and assist those who might be motivated to stop AAS abuse.

DETECTION OF ANABOLIC ANDROGENIC STEROID USE

Due to concerns for the rampant use of AASs among elite athletes, WADA and other antidoping agencies have been updating their testing practices and expanding the list of banned substances. A longitudinal monitoring program called the biological passport has recently been developed to prevent and detect the use of performance-enhancing drugs. The basic premise is to establish a "baseline" profile of various urinary androgen precursors and metabolites and then evaluating for changes in these urinary compounds over time. WADA has outlined detailed methodologies on how testing of elite athletes should be performed, and these are well-outlined in a prior publication.[21] Assays for various androgens and their metabolites have been continually modified over time to improve sensitivity and accuracy. Athletes tend to use many evasive techniques such as dilution, using someone else's urine sample or providing a sample from a time when they are not using AAS to avoid detection. To circumvent this, strict guidelines have been implemented for testing athletes, including testing at random times, and even observed micturition.

The approach to detecting AAS abuse in clinical practice differs (**Fig. 2**). Clinicians should suspect AAS abuse in a muscular man who presents with concerns of infertility, gynecomastia, or evaluation for testosterone supplementation. These men might report a decline or plateau in their strength or muscle bulk when training with weights and usually have "bigorexia" or muscular dysmorphia, a distorted body image that they are not muscular enough.[22] Physical examination reveals a normal virilization and large or hypertrophic muscles. When serum luteinizing hormone (LH) is suppressed to the lower limit of detection, testicular volumes are usually reduced by 25% to 35%.[23] However, if the baseline testicular volumes were 25 cc or greater, then the AAS abuser will not have "small testes." Testicular texture (softness) is not useful. Gynecomastia or breast tenderness can be another clinical finding in men who use aromatizable nontestosterone androgens or androgen precursors that disproportionately raise serum estradiol concentrations compared with testosterone.

Initial hormonal evaluation should include the measurement of serum testosterone, follicle-stimulating hormone (FSH), and LH. Interpretation of these laboratories is summarized in **Table 2**. It is not useful to measure urinary precursors or metabolites of androgens in clinical practice. First, these assays are not widely available in commercial

Table 1
Agents that are commonly used for anabolic androgenic steroid abuse

Exogenous Androgens (Generic/Common Name)	
"Designer Androgens"	*Endogenous Androgens Used as Drugs*
Bolandiol	Testosterone
Clostebol (Steranobol)	Dihydrotestosterone
Danazol	Boldenone (Equipoise)
Drostanolone (Masteron)	Nandrolone (Durabolin)
Gestrinone	
Metandienone (Dianabol)	
Metenolone (Primabolan)	
Oxandrolone (Anavar)	
Oxymetholone (Anadrol)	
Stanozolol (Winstrol)	
Tetrahydrogestrinone (The Clear)	
Trenbolone (Trenabol)	
Androgen Precursors	
Androstenedione (Andro)	
Androsterone	
Dehydroepiandrostenedione (DHEA)	
Gonadotropins	
hCG	
Recombinant human LH	
Aromatase inhibitors	
Anastrozole	
Letrozole	
Exemestane	
Selective estrogen receptor modulators	
Clomiphene	
Raloxifene	

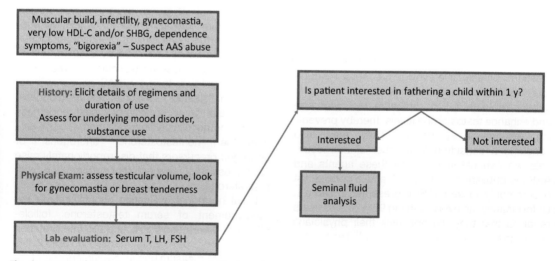

Fig. 2. Proposed initial evaluation when AAS abuse is suspected. This figure depicts an approach to the initial evaluation of a patient with AAS abuse or suspected AAS abuse. AASs, anabolic androgenic steroids; HDL-C, high density lipoprotein cholesterol; SHBG, sex-hormone binding globulin.

Table 2
Clinical signs and serum hormone concentrations during anabolic androgenic steroid use

Agent Used	New Onset or Tender Gynecomastia	Testes <15 cc	Serum Testosterone	Serum FSH	Serum LH
Testosterone	More common	More common	↑	↓	↓
Nontestosterone androgenic steroids	More common[a]	More common	↓	↓	↓
Testosterone precursors[b]	More common	More common	↑	↓	↓
Gonadotropins (eg, hCG)	Common	No	↑	↓	↓
Aromatase inhibitor alone	Uncommon	No	↑	↑	↑
SERM (eg, clomiphene)	?	No	↑	↑	↑

Abbreviations: FSH, follicle stimulating hormone; hCG, human chorionic gonadotropin; LH, luteinizing hormone; SERM, selective estrogen receptor modulator.
[a] If agent is aromatizable.
[b] Symptoms manifest only at very high dosages.

laboratories for individual patients. Second, it is not possible to prevent submission of a urine sample during a time of nonuse or substitute a urine sample from a nonuser. Subsequent discussion with patients entails a discussion about the potential for adverse effects with a long-term AAS use and possible options to taper off.

ADVERSE EFFECTS OF ANABOLIC ANDROGENIC STEROID ABUSE

Is the use of AAS harmful? This question cannot be answered simply because it depends on the agent used, route of administration, dose and duration of use, use of adjunctive therapies and substances, and a person's age and underlying physical and mental health. Some adverse effects are class effects of androgens, such as suppressive effects on the hypothalamic-pituitary-testicular axis and erythrocytosis but other effects are specific such as hepatotoxicity with oral alkylated testosterone derivatives. Use of nonaromatizable androgens and aromatase inhibitors might have a higher likelihood of causing reductions in libido or erectile function due to the decreased estradiol production.[24] Changes in high-density lipoprotein-cholesterol (HDL-C) are more notable with oral formulations. Sporadic or transient use of AAS is less likely to have lasting adverse impacts on health; however, there are some data to support long-term effects of chronic high dose AAS use. Unfortunately, the data are weak and derived from case reports and series, case-control studies, and cross-sectional studies. In the following sections, we will review

the potential adverse effects (**Fig. 3**) and the strength of the data for causation for each adverse effect (**Table 3**).

Reproductive Function

The use of an exogenous androgen exerts negative feedback inhibition at the hypothalamus and pituitary glands via the androgen and estrogen receptors and results in suppression of endogenous testosterone and sperm production.[25,26] Although using an AAS, its androgen action is sufficient to prevent hypogonadal symptoms (fatigue, decreased libido, erectile dysfunction) but these symptoms can develop in between cycles of use when the hypothalamic-pituitary-testicular axis is still suppressed. Aromatizable androgens, particularly at high doses, and hCG therapy (that stimulates aromatase) can cause tender gynecomastia. Some AASs are not aromatized; otherwise, men might use aromatase inhibitors (to avoid gynecomastia) that can lower estradiol concentrations considerably. In this setting, low serum estradiol concentrations can result in decrease in libido or erectile dysfunction despite androgenic effects of the AASs.[24] Many AAS abusers will detect testicular shrinkage over time but not men who use hCG. The timeline of recovery for the hypothalamic-pituitary-gonadal axis can be months[27] or years,[28,29] depending on duration and dosage of AAS use. In some men who have abused high dosages for years, the suppression of the gonadal axis may persist for many years (or indefinitely).[30] Additionally, in men who

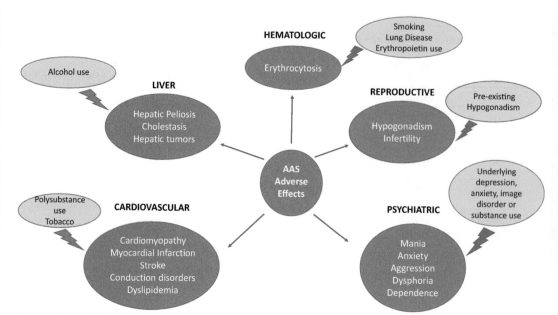

Fig. 3. Adverse effects of AAS abuse by system. This figure outlines the various known or suspected adverse effects of AAS use (in blue) and the potential confounding factors (in orange) that could exacerbate or be the primary cause of the adverse effect. AAS, anabolic androgenic steroids.

do not recover their gonadal function within 1 year after cessation of AAS use, the possibility of underlying classic causes of hypogonadism should be considered (eg, pituitary macroadenoma or Klinefelter syndrome). Men can present with infertility due to the inhibition of spermatogenesis, during or long after AAS abuse. Therefore, the abuse of AAS can cause variable presentations (see **Table 2**).[31–35] Depending on the regimen used, symptoms may develop during a cycle, in between cycles (for short-acting AASs), or persist after cessation of use.

Psychiatric Disturbances

Several psychiatric symptoms have been reported with AAS use, with certain symptoms developing during use while others constitute a "withdrawal syndrome." In studies of the psychiatric impact of AASs, investigators have interviewed AAS users about their psychiatric history "on" and "off" drug,[36–39] whereas other investigators have compared AAS users with nonusers using structured interviews and psychological scales[40–45] or followed AAS users longitudinally with

Table 3
Studies on adverse systemic effects of anabolic androgenic steroid use

Adverse Effect	Case Report/Series	Cohort Study or Case-Control Study	Cross-Sectional Study	Clinical Trials	Other (Meta-Analyses)
Reproductive function	212,213,28,29,30	27	31,32		33,34
Psychiatric disturbances	37,38,43,46,49	36,39,40,41,42,44,45,47		3,54,55,56,57	
Cardiovascular Effects	60,61,62,63,64,65,66,67,68,69,70, 71,72,73,74,75,76,77,78,79,80, 81,82,83,84,85,86,87,88,89,91,104	90,92,93,94,95,96,97, 98,100,105,106		101,102	
Hepatic Effects	110,114,115,118,119,120		113,117		109
Erythrocytosis	77,133,134	105		125,126,127, 129,131,132	128,130

The numbers in the various cells represent the reference number of the study demonstrating each adverse effect.

assessments during "on" and "off" cycles.[46,47] There seems to be a dose-related effect of AASs on mood disorders, particularly at doses equivalent or higher than 1000 mg testosterone per week.[5,48] There are also numerous observational reports that describe uncharacteristically aggressive or violent behaviors in previously normal individuals[5,49] who are using AASs. There have also been studies of supraphysiologic androgen exposure in healthy men using 300 mg of testosterone enanthate per week that demonstrated no adverse psychiatric effects[50–53] but this dosage is not comparable with those used by many chronic AAS abusers (500–1000 mg or greater per week). Placebo-controlled studies of the effects of 500 mg per week of testosterone[3,54–57] showed that 4.6% of men had hypomanic or manic symptoms compared with none on placebo. Based on the observational data from AAS abusers and experimental studies of high doses of testosterone in healthy men, there seems to be biological plausibility for a causal role of androgens in the reported psychiatric manifestations in a minority of AAS users. Symptoms that have been described during AAS abuse encompass issues with impulse control, aggression, anxiety, hypomania, and mania. When "off" the AAS agents, mainly depressive symptoms can develop—depressed mood, apathy, hypersomnia, anorexia, loss of libido, suicidality—that are likely due to a combination of sudden withdrawal of supraphysiologic androgen action as well as clinical hypogonadism. Potential confounders in all these presentations include underlying psychiatric disorders such as anxiety and depression[58,59] and concurrent use and abuse of alcohol and/or illicit drugs.

Cardiovascular Effects

Various adverse cardiovascular effects have been described in case reports and series from AAS use. These comprise cardiomyopathy,[60–65] myocardial infarction,[66–77] cerebrovascular accidents,[78–80] conduction abnormalities,[81–84] and coagulation abnormalities.[70,85–89] Evidence of cardiomyopathy has also been shown from postmortem studies showing greater cardiac mass[90] and ventricular hypertrophy with fibrosis[91] in AAS users; echocardiography[92–99] and cardiac MRI[100] have demonstrated decreased ventricular ejection fractions and reduced diastolic tissue velocities.

The best-defined adverse effect of AAS use on cardiovascular risk is a reduction in HDL-C, particularly with oral formulations.[101–103] However, whether this dyslipidemia increases atherosclerotic events is unclear although one study did report considerably higher coronary artery calcium

scores than expected for men of that age in 14 professional weightlifters with long-term AAS use history.[104] A 2022 cohort study of 100 AAS abusers demonstrated reductions in HDL-C, apoprotein A and lipoprotein (a) and an increase in low-density lipoprotein-cholesterol, and apoprotein B.[105] Another cohort study of 86 weightlifters with a long-term AAS use showed myocardial dysfunction and accelerated atherosclerosis.[106] A limitation of these data is confounding from the high prevalence of tobacco and illicit substance use (cocaine, amphetamines) among these populations[107,108] but a sensitivity analysis looking at the contribution of these factors did not change their outcomes significantly.[106]

Hepatic System

A common misconception is that AAS use causes hepatotoxicity; however, this adverse effect is seen only with oral 17α-alkylated androgens.[109–112] The main consequences that have been described include hepatic peliosis[113–115] (a condition in which blood-filled cysts accumulate in the liver), cholestasis,[113] and various types of hepatic tumors.[109,115–120] One potential confounding factor is the development of transaminase elevations from excessive exercise in AAS users can be mistaken for hepatotoxicity.[121]

Erythrocytosis

Androgens have a stimulating effect on erythropoiesis through multiple possible mechanisms: increasing sensitivity to erythropoietin, suppressing hepcidin transcription and increasing iron availability to erythrocytes.[122–124] The use of AASs has been associated with dose-related increases in hemoglobin and hematocrit. This has been shown in clinical trials of healthy men treated with supraphysiologic doses of testosterone,[125–129] hypogonadal older men,[130–132] and in case reports of AAS abusers.[77,133,134] A recent cohort study of AAS abusers (n = 100) that followed them around the time of use as well as thereafter, showed a mean absolute increase in hematocrit of 3%, which was transient and normalized shortly after cessation of use (at 3 months and 1 year).[105] Potential confounders could include the use of other performance-enhancing techniques (abuse of erythropoietin or blood transfusions) or concurrent long-standing smoking history resulting in chronic obstructive pulmonary disease and hypoxemia. The concern with increasing red blood cell mass is the potential risk of increased viscosity of blood and its effects on cardiovascular disease. Studies have linked an elevated hematocrit to a higher rate of cardiovascular death,[135] cerebral infarction,[136–138] and coronary heart disease.[139–143] However, the data linking AAS-use-induced erythrocytosis to adverse cardiovascular events is anecdotal.

Other Adverse Effects

Several other adverse effects of AAS abuse have also been described. Among musculoskeletal effects, tendon ruptures[144,145] and rhabdomyolysis[146,147] have been noted. The evidence of increased risk of tendon ruptures is based on case reports, and proposed mechanisms include disproportionate strength of hypertrophied muscles[148] as well as deleterious effects of AAS on the architecture of tendons,[149,150] as seen in preclinical models. Similarly, multiple case reports of rhabdomyolysis exist and is likely related to the excessive exercise that AAS abusers tend to engage in. Chronic effects of high doses of androgens on the pilosebaceous units can result in acne and androgenic alopecia.[151] Chronic kidney disease[152,153] has been described in a case report and case series with AAS abuse. There is an expected increase in serum creatinine in these users due to muscle hypertrophy. However, proteinuria and glomerulosclerosis have been described[153] and hypothesized to be due to a combination of postadaptive glomerular changes secondary to increased lean body mass and direct nephrotoxic effects of AAS. Finally, AAS abuse is associated with higher risk for various infections.[19,154,155] These include blood-borne infections such as HIV, hepatitis B and C, as well as skin and soft-tissue infections from unclean injection practices. In an Internet survey, 13% of AAS abusers admitted to unsafe needle practices.[12] Other risk factors that predispose AAS abusers to infections such as HIV, hepatitis B and C, include the high rate of use of these agents among homosexual[156] and incarcerated men.[157–159]

To summarize, in men, AAS abuse leads to suppression of testosterone and sperm production that is generally reversible within 1 to 2 years but the recovery time depends on duration, dose, and half-life of the AAS. There is also a dose-dependent increase in hematocrit that might lead to frank erythrocytosis. In some men, high dosages of AASs might cause psychiatric disturbances. Cessation after prolonged abuse of AAS is associated with a withdrawal syndrome that includes depression and fatigue and can be difficult to distinguish from persistent suppression of the hypothalamic-pituitary-testicular axis. There is an association between AAS abuse and cardiovascular disease that is concerning but this association is influenced by confounders such as a high prevalence of tobacco use, cocaine, amphetamines, and poor health habits in AAS abusers.

MANAGEMENT OF ANABOLIC ANDROGENIC STEROID USE AMONG THE GENERAL POPULATION

As reviewed before, some people use AAS fleetingly in their lifetime and can escape any lasting consequences of such an exposure. However, among those who develop dependence to these agents, clinical pathways for management are not well established. The initial assessment by medical professionals (see **Fig. 2**) should include evaluating whether the patient has dependence symptoms such as dysphoria, depression, fatigue, loss of libido or body (muscular) dysmorphia when not using AAS. Eliciting what the patient's motivations for ongoing use are and the presence of any associated history of depression, anxiety, and substance use issues are extremely important. Having a frank discussion about the duration and nature of AAS use and assessing the patient's readiness to stop using are the essential first steps in building trust with the patient and laying the framework to make any recommendations in the future (**Fig. 4**). It is also important to assess their near-term goals for their health and fertility (see **Fig. 4**).

Men Unwilling to Stop Anabolic Androgenic Steroid Use

For men who are not ready to quit AAS use, offering the option of prescription testosterone therapy, sometimes at supraphysiologic dose (such as testosterone cypionate 150 mg intramuscularly every week or more) can help build a physician–patient relationship that opens the door to closer monitoring for side effects and facilitates tapered discontinuation of AAS use.[22] Prescription testosterone therapy is safer than continued nonprescription AAS abuse because unregulated sources of androgens are often contaminated with miscellaneous compounds.

Men Willing to Stop Anabolic Androgenic Steroid Use

When men are interested in quitting AAS use, there are no FDA-approved treatment options, and the management approach largely depends on the person's fertility goals and duration of use.

Men desiring to father a pregnancy within 1 year

For men who wish to conceive within the next ~12 months, a seminal fluid analysis should be performed. Ideally, 2 seminal fluid samples

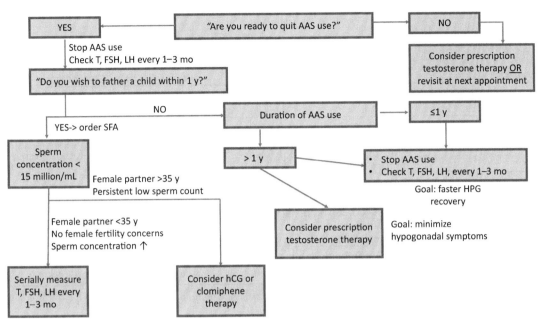

Fig. 4. Proposed discussion of cessation of AAS use, fertility needs and treatment options with patient. This figure outlines a suggested algorithm to assess a patient's readiness to quit AAS abuse and to assess their fertility goals. AASs, anabolic androgenic steroids; FSH, follicle stimulating hormone; hCG, human chorionic gonadotropin; HPG, hypothalamic-pituitary-gonadal; LH, luteinizing hormone; SFA, seminal fluid analysis; T, testosterone.

obtained after 2 to 7 days of ejaculatory abstinence should be analyzed. The time to recovery of the hypothalamic-pituitary-gonadal axis varies based on duration and route of AAS use, and it can be months[27] or years.[28,29] For those who have been using AAS for considerably longer than 1 to 2 years, the recovery is slower and requires longer term monitoring. This unpredictable recovery time of the hypothalamic-pituitary-gonadal axis may not align with their reproductive timeline and goals. This becomes particularly relevant if the female partner in the relationship is older (35 years or above) or also has infertility issues. In such men, the use of agents such as hCG[29] or clomiphene[160,161] have been described (**Table 4**), if their semen concentration is low. There are very little data to support effectiveness of hCG or clomiphene in men who have stopped AAS abuse. It is our recommendation to consider hCG therapy over clomiphene due to the lack of any safety concerns. Clomiphene is a SERM, which increases serum gonadotropins and testosterone concentrations within 2 to 4 weeks in men with intact hypothalamic-pituitary-gonadal function.[162–164] Although doses up to 100 mg every other day have not revealed adverse events in men aged younger than 50 years in these short-term studies, there are case reports of venous thromboembolism associated with clomiphene use by

men.[165,166] hCG has the biological activity of LH and stimulated the Leydig cells in the testes to make testosterone. The increase in intratesticular testosterone drives spermatogenesis.[167] On hCG therapy, serum testosterone is monitored every 1 to 2 months, with the goal of achieving concentrations of 400 to 800 ng/dL. Subsequently, sperm concentrations are assessed every 1 to 3 months, with the goal of achieving at least 5 to 10 million sperm/mL of ejaculate and/or pregnancy. However, hCG increases testosterone while keeping gonadotropins suppressed. So, if after 6 months of hCG therapy, there has been an insufficient sperm response or lack of pregnancy, addition of FSH (either as human menopausal gonadotropin, or recombinant human FSH) can be considered to stimulated spermatogenesis. There are no safety concerns with hCG when used at dosages that maintain serum testosterone concentrations in the normal range. New onset of gynecomastia occurs in some men because the LH activity of hCG increases aromatization of testosterone to estradiol. A discussion with the patient is required, outlining a treatment plan of a 12 to 24-month trial (see **Table 4**) of these options, to increase serum testosterone in the upper half of normal range to see if it stimulates spermatogenesis, while acknowledging the unknown risks and likelihood of success.

Table 4
Proposed trial for induction of spermatogenesis in infertile men with prior anabolic androgenic steroid use with near-term fertility goals

Agent	Clomiphene	Human Chorionic Gonadotropin
Starting Dose	25 mg orally every other day	1000–2000 IU subcutaneously 2–3 times a week
Dose escalation	Increase by 12.5–25 mg every other day on monthly basis if serum testosterone less than the lower limit of normal	Increase weekly dosage by 1000–2000 IU on monthly basis if serum testosterone less than the lower limit of normal
Maximum	100 mg every other day	4000–6000 IU 2–3 times a week
Monitoring	Serum T, FSH and LH every month Once T in 400–800 ng/dL range for 3–6 mo, measure sperm concentration	Serum T every month Once T in 400–800 ng/dL range for 3–6 mo, measure sperm concentration
Side Effects	Venous thromboembolism	Injection site discomfort, cost
Outcomes	Anecdotal success in case reports	Anecdotal success in case reports

Abbreviations: AAS, anabolic androgenic steroids; IU, international units; ng/dL, nanograms per deciliter; T, testosterone.

No immediate desire for fertility

For men who have used AASs for less than a year duration, AAS can be stopped, and they can be monitored approximately every 3 months with assessment of serum testosterone and gonadotropins. Assessment of a seminal fluid analysis might never be required or can at least be deferred until after serum testosterone return to the normal range for 3 to 6 months. While waiting for the hypothalamic-pituitary-gonadal axis to recover, prescription testosterone therapy can be considered to ameliorate severe symptoms of hypogonadism but men should be counseled that this will maintain the suppression of serum endogenous gonadotropins, testosterone, and spermatogenesis.

POTENTIAL CLINICAL USES OF PRESCRIPTION ANDROGENS

AAS abuse is distinct from testosterone pharmacotherapy in men with hypogonadism. Diagnosing hypogonadism (primary or secondary) in a symptomatic patient with unequivocally low serum testosterone concentrations and appropriate treatment with testosterone therapy is not controversial and is the accepted standard of care.[168] Treating middle-aged to older men with borderline serum testosterone concentrations without convincing hypogonadal symptoms with physiologic doses of testosterone has been increasing. Reviewing the risks and benefits of such therapy and its appropriateness is not the aim of our current article, and we direct the readers to recent reviews.[169–171] There might be

a role of AAS beyond testosterone replacement therapy for hypogonadism. In this section, we will summarize studies that have explored nontraditional uses of AAS.

Muscle-Wasting Conditions

Androgens are anabolic. Historically, these were measured in animal models by calculating the ratio of the change in levator ani weight (muscle-building or anabolic effect) to change in ventral prostate weight (androgenic effect).[172] Agents such as testosterone, dihydrotestosterone, and methyltestosterone have an anabolic to androgenic action ratio of about 1:1. However, other androgens, such as oxandrolone and nandrolone, have a ratio that is closer to 10:1[173,174] and have significant myotrophic effects. As such, these and other androgens have been used in severe catabolic states that cause muscle-wasting such as severe burns,[175,176] HIV/acquired immunodeficiency syndrome-associated wasting,[177–180] hemodialysis,[181] neuromuscular diseases such as Duchenne muscular dystrophy,[182–184] amyotrophic lateral sclerosis,[185] chronic obstructive pulmonary disease (COPD),[186–189] and protein catabolism from chronic corticosteroid therapy.[190] These studies have demonstrated measurable improvements in bone mineral content, total body weight, and lean body mass as well as reduction in hospital and rehabilitation facility lengths of stay. One important consideration is the possibility of coexisting hypogonadism in these chronic disease states and the need to evaluate such patients appropriately and treat when indicated.

Hypoproliferative Anemias

As previously mentioned, androgens have a stimulant effect on erythropoiesis.[122–124] This action has been used to treat a variety of anemias. In patients with aplastic anemia, various androgens have been investigated with and without corticosteroids[191–193] and response rates have varied from 40% to 100%.[194–196] Among patients with anemia due to chronic kidney disease, various androgens have been investigated with and without erythropoietin therapy[197–199] and have shown an increase in erythropoietin levels[200] and hemoglobin,[201] as well as reduction[201] or even elimination[202] of transfusion needs. Androgens have also been studied in treatment of other anemias including refractory anemias, anemia from chronic lymphocytic leukemia and hemolytic anemia with success.[193] Despite their clear beneficial effects on erythropoiesis in various anemic states, their use remains controversial due to concerns for development of androgenic side effects, polycythemia, and concerns for cardiovascular risks. Therefore, at this time, androgen therapy is considered second-line therapy or adjunctive to erythropoietin.

Male Hormonal Contraception

Androgens have been studied as hormonal contraceptive methods in men for many decades now. Studies using testosterone have proven effective at preventing pregnancies with greater than 95% efficacy, alone or in combination with progestins in various contraceptive efficacy trials.[203–208] These regimens have faced challenges such as inconvenient dosing regimens (weekly injections) and notable adverse effects (acne, modest weight gain, reduction in HDL-C, mood changes), which have hampered any product from coming to market. Novel androgens such as dimethandrolone undecanoate[209] and 11β-methyl-19-nortestosterone dodecylcarbonate[210] are being studied as potential daily oral or long-acting injectable formulations for male contraception. Another regimen that is currently undergoing an efficacy trial is a daily topical novel progestin, nestorone, formulated as a combined gel with testosterone.[211] If these agents move forward in drug development, they could revolutionize the world of contraception, distributing the burden more evenly among the sexes.

SUMMARY

The use of AASs is prevalent among the international athletic community. Although young male body builders are more likely to use AASs, it is unclear how common chronic AAS abuse is in the general population. Among those who abuse high dosages, infertility, erythrocytosis, neuropsychiatric adverse effects are the most common adverse effects. AAS abuse might also increase cardiovascular risk. There are no established care pathways to detect and treat patients who have abused AASs. Frank, respectful discussion with the patient is the best approach. The main approved indication for therapeutic use of AASs is for male hypogonadism. However, other novel uses of these agents include muscle-wasting conditions, anemias, and male hormonal contraception. A better understanding of the breadth and magnitude of the long-term effects of AAS on various organ systems by means of clinical trials will further our ability to manage their use among athletes and the public, as well as optimize their use in various disease states.

CLINICS CARE POINTS

- The possibility of androgenic steroid use should be considered in men who exhibit muscle hypertrophy, particularly if associated with infertility.
- Laboratory clues include elevated hemoglobin/hematocrit, low high-density lipoprotein-cholesterol (HDL-C) and low sex-hormone binding globulin (SHBG).
- Hormone assessment demonstrates suppressed serum gonadotropins (follicle-stimulating hormone and luteinizing hormone) and low serum testosterone, if abusing non-testosterone androgens, or high-normal to high serum testosterone, if abusing testosterone precursors or drugs with luteinizing hormone activity such as human chorionic gonadotropin (hCG).
- Clomiphene use results in a distinct pattern of high-normal to high gonadotropins and high serum testosterone without suppression of HDL-C or low SHBG.
- The topic of discontinuation of use is best approached in a nonjudgmental manner by educating them about long-term adverse consequences.
- There is not any recommended approach to helping men wean off anabolic androgenic steroid regimens but prescription of modestly higher than replacement dosages of testosterone followed by a tapering of the dosage might be effective and prevent loss to follow-up. If duration of abuse was less than 1 year, it is reasonable to recommend discontinuation of androgenic steroid abuse

without prescription of testosterone therapy. Most men who have abused androgenic steroids for less than 1 year will recover serum testosterone and gonadotropins to normal within 1 to 2 months.

DISCLOSURE

A. Thirumalai and B.D. Anawalt: Nothing to disclose.

REFERENCES

1. Nieschlag E, Nieschlag S. ENDOCRINE HISTORY: The history of discovery, synthesis and development of testosterone for clinical use. Eur J Endocrinol 2019;180(6):R201–12.
2. Fitch KD. Androgenic-anabolic steroids and the Olympic Games. Asian J Androl 2008;10(3): 384–90.
3. Bhasin S, Storer TW, Berman N, et al. The effects of supraphysiologic doses of testosterone on muscle size and strength in normal men. N Engl J Med 1996;335(1):1–7.
4. Sagoe D, Molde H, Andreassen CS, et al. The global epidemiology of anabolic-androgenic steroid use: a meta-analysis and meta-regression analysis. Ann Epidemiol 2014;24(5):383–98.
5. Bhasin S, Hatfield DL, Hoffman JR, et al. Anabolic-Androgenic Steroid Use in Sports, Health, and Society. Med Sci Sports Exerc 2021;53(8):1778–94.
6. Pope HG, Kanayama G, Ionescu-Pioggia M, et al. Anabolic steroid users' attitudes towards physicians. Addiction 2004;99(9):1189–94.
7. Morente-Sanchez J, Zabala M. Doping in sport: a review of elite athletes' attitudes, beliefs, and knowledge. Sports Med 2013;43(6):395–411.
8. Hoffman JR, Kraemer WJ, Bhasin S, et al. Position stand on androgen and human growth hormone use. J Strength Cond Res 2009;23(5 Suppl):S1–59.
9. Kersey RD, Elliot DL, Goldberg L, et al. National Athletic Trainers' Association position statement: anabolic-androgenic steroids. J Athl Train 2012; 47(5):567–88.
10. Perry PJ, Lund BC, Deninger MJ, et al. Anabolic steroid use in weightlifters and bodybuilders: an internet survey of drug utilization. Clin J Sport Med 2005;15(5):326–30.
11. Santos AM, da Rocha MS, da Silva MF. Illicit use and abuse of anabolic-androgenic steroids among Brazilian bodybuilders. Subst Use Misuse 2011; 46(6):742–8.
12. Pope HG Jr, Wood RI, Rogol A, et al. Adverse health consequences of performance-enhancing drugs: an Endocrine Society scientific statement. Endocr Rev 2014;35(3):341–75.
13. Pope HG Jr, Kanayama G, Athey A, et al. The lifetime prevalence of anabolic-androgenic steroid use and dependence in Americans: current best estimates. Am J Addict 2014;23(4):371–7.
14. Hakansson A, Mickelsson K, Wallin C, et al. Anabolic androgenic steroids in the general population: user characteristics and associations with substance use. Eur Addict Res 2012;18(2):83–90.
15. LaBotz M, Griesemer BA, Council On Sports M, et al. Use of Performance-Enhancing Substances. Pediatrics 2016;138(1).
16. Kann L, Kinchen S, Shanklin SL, et al. Youth risk behavior surveillance–United States, 2013. MMWR Suppl 2014;63(4):1–168.
17. Hildebrandt T, Langenbucher JW, Carr SJ, et al. Modeling population heterogeneity in appearance- and performance-enhancing drug (APED) use: applications of mixture modeling in 400 regular APED users. J Abnorm Psychol 2007;116(4):717–33.
18. Zahnow R, McVeigh J, Bates G, et al. Identifying a typology of men who use anabolic androgenic steroids (AAS). Int J Drug Policy 2018;55:105–12.
19. Ip EJ, Barnett MJ, Tenerowicz MJ, et al. The Anabolic 500 survey: characteristics of male users versus nonusers of anabolic-androgenic steroids for strength training. Pharmacotherapy 2011; 31(8):757–66.
20. Cohen J, Collins R, Darkes J, et al. A league of their own: demographics, motivations and patterns of use of 1,955 male adult non-medical anabolic steroid users in the United States. J Int Soc Sports Nutr 2007;4:12.
21. Anawalt BD. Detection of anabolic androgenic steroid use by elite athletes and by members of the general public. Mol Cell Endocrinol 2018;464:21–7.
22. Anawalt BD. Diagnosis and Management of Anabolic Androgenic Steroid Use. J Clin Endocrinol Metab 2019;104(7):2490–500.
23. Anawalt BD, Amory JK, Herbst KL, et al. Intramuscular testosterone enanthate plus very low dosage oral levonorgestrel suppresses spermatogenesis without causing weight gain in normal young men: a randomized clinical trial. J Androl 2005; 26(3):405–13.
24. Finkelstein JS, Yu EW, Burnett-Bowie SA. Gonadal steroids and body composition, strength, and sexual function in men. New Engl J Med 2013;369(25): 2457.
25. Tan RS, Scally MC. Anabolic steroid-induced hypogonadism–towards a unified hypothesis of anabolic steroid action. Med Hypotheses 2009; 72(6):723–8.
26. Reyes-Fuentes A, Veldhuis JD. Neuroendocrine physiology of the normal male gonadal axis. Endocrinol Metab Clin North Am 1993;22(1):93–124.
27. Garevik N, Strahm E, Garle M, et al. Long term perturbation of endocrine parameters and

cholesterol metabolism after discontinued abuse of anabolic androgenic steroids. J Steroid Biochem Mol Biol 2011;127(3–5):295–300.

28. van Breda E, Keizer HA, Kuipers H, et al. Androgenic anabolic steroid use and severe hypothalamic-pituitary dysfunction: a case study. Int J Sports Med 2003;24(3):195–6.

29. Menon DK. Successful treatment of anabolic steroid-induced azoospermia with human chorionic gonadotropin and human menopausal gonadotropin. Fertil Steril 2003;79(Suppl 3):1659–61.

30. Boregowda K, Joels L, Stephens JW, et al. Persistent primary hypogonadism associated with anabolic steroid abuse. Fertil Steril 2011;96(1): e7–8.

31. Kanayama G, Hudson JI, DeLuca J, et al. Prolonged hypogonadism in males following withdrawal from anabolic-androgenic steroids: an under-recognized problem. Addiction 2015; 110(5):823–31.

32. Rasmussen JJ, Selmer C, Ostergren PB, et al. Former Abusers of Anabolic Androgenic Steroids Exhibit Decreased Testosterone Levels and Hypogonadal Symptoms Years after Cessation: A Case-Control Study. PLoS One 2016;11(8): e0161208.

33. Christou MA, Christou PA, Markozannes G, et al. Effects of Anabolic Androgenic Steroids on the Reproductive System of Athletes and Recreational Users: A Systematic Review and Meta-Analysis. Sports Med 2017;47(9):1869–83.

34. Rahnema CD, Lipshultz LI, Crosnoe LE, et al. Anabolic steroid-induced hypogonadism: diagnosis and treatment. Fertil Steril 2014;101(5): 1271–9.

35. Vilar Neto JO, da Silva CA, Bruno da Silva CA, et al. Anabolic androgenic steroid-induced hypogonadism, a reversible condition in male individuals? A systematic review. Andrologia 2021;53(7):e14062.

36. Pope HG Jr, Katz DL. Psychiatric and medical effects of anabolic-androgenic steroid use. A controlled study of 160 athletes. Arch Gen Psychiatry 1994;51(5):375–82.

37. Pope HG Jr, Katz DL. Affective and psychotic symptoms associated with anabolic steroid use. Am J Psychiatry 1988;145(4):487–90.

38. Parrott AC, Choi PY, Davies M. Anabolic steroid use by amateur athletes: effects upon psychological mood states. J Sports Med Phys Fitness 1994;34(3):292–8.

39. Cooper CJ, Noakes TD, Dunne T, et al. A high prevalence of abnormal personality traits in chronic users of anabolic-androgenic steroids. Br J Sports Med 1996;30(3):246–50.

40. Bahrke MS, Wright JE, Strauss RH, et al. Psychological moods and subjectively perceived behavioral and somatic changes accompanying anabolic-androgenic steroid use. Am J Sports Med 1992;20(6):717–24.

41. Midgley SJ, Heather N, Davies JB. Levels of aggression among a group of anabolic-androgenic steroid users. Med Sci Law 2001; 41(4):309–14.

42. Choi PY, Pope HG Jr. Violence toward women and illicit androgenic-anabolic steroid use. Ann Clin Psychiatry 1994;6(1):21–5.

43. Perry PJ, Andersen KH, Yates WR. Illicit anabolic steroid use in athletes. A case series analysis. Am J Sports Med 1990;18(4):422–8.

44. Perry PJ, Kutscher EC, Lund BC, et al. Measures of aggression and mood changes in male weightlifters with and without androgenic anabolic steroid use. J Forensic Sci 2003;48(3):646–51.

45. Yates WR, Perry P, Murray S. Aggression and hostility in anabolic steroid users. Biol Psychiatry 1992; 31(12):1232–4.

46. Fudala PJ, Weinrieb RM, Calarco JS, et al. An evaluation of anabolic-androgenic steroid abusers over a period of 1 year: seven case studies. Ann Clin Psychiatry 2003;15(2):121–30.

47. Pagonis TA, Angelopoulos NV, Koukoulis GN, et al. Psychiatric side effects induced by supraphysiological doses of combinations of anabolic steroids correlate to the severity of abuse. Eur Psychiatry 2006;21(8):551–62.

48. Onakomaiya MM, Henderson LP. Mad men, women and steroid cocktails: a review of the impact of sex and other factors on anabolic androgenic steroids effects on affective behaviors. Psychopharmacology (Berl) 2016;233(4):549–69.

49. Pope HG Jr, Kanayama G, Hudson JI, et al. Review Article: Anabolic-Androgenic Steroids, Violence, and Crime: Two Cases and Literature Review. Am J Addict 2021;30(5):423–32.

50. Friedl KE, Dettori JR, Hannan CJ Jr, et al. Comparison of the effects of high dose testosterone and 19-nortestosterone to a replacement dose of testosterone on strength and body composition in normal men. J Steroid Biochem Mol Biol 1991; 40(4–6):607–12.

51. Friedl KE, Jones RE, Hannan CJ Jr, et al. The administration of pharmacological doses of testosterone or 19-nortestosterone to normal men is not associated with increased insulin secretion or impaired glucose tolerance. J Clin Endocrinol Metab 1989;68(5):971–5.

52. Hannan CJ Jr, Friedl KE, Zold A, et al. Psychological and serum homovanillic acid changes in men administered androgenic steroids. Psychoneuroendocrinology 1991;16(4):335–43.

53. Matsumoto AM. Effects of chronic testosterone administration in normal men: safety and efficacy of high dosage testosterone and parallel dose-dependent suppression of luteinizing hormone,

follicle-stimulating hormone, and sperm production. J Clin Endocrinol Metab 1990;70(1):282–7.

54. Pope HG Jr, Kouri EM, Hudson JI. Effects of supraphysiologic doses of testosterone on mood and aggression in normal men: a randomized controlled trial. Arch Gen Psychiatry 2000;57(2): 133–40 [discussion: 155–6].

55. Su TP, Pagliaro M, Schmidt PJ, et al. Neuropsychiatric effects of anabolic steroids in male normal volunteers. JAMA 1993;269(21):2760–4.

56. Tricker R, Casaburi R, Storer TW, et al. The effects of supraphysiological doses of testosterone on angry behavior in healthy eugonadal men–a clinical research center study. J Clin Endocrinol Metab 1996;81(10):3754–8.

57. Yates WR, Perry PJ, MacIndoe J, et al. Psychosexual effects of three doses of testosterone cycling in normal men. Biol Psychiatry 1999; 45(3):254–60.

58. Bahrke MS, Yesalis CE 3rd. Weight training. A potential confounding factor in examining the psychological and behavioural effects of anabolic-androgenic steroids. Sports Med 1994;18(5): 309–18.

59. Bahrke MS, Yesalis CE 3rd, Wright JE. Psychological and behavioural effects of endogenous testosterone and anabolic-androgenic steroids. An update. Sports Med 1996;22(6):367–90.

60. Clark BM, Schofield RS. Dilated cardiomyopathy and acute liver injury associated with combined use of ephedra, gamma-hydroxybutyrate, and anabolic steroids. Pharmacotherapy 2005;25(5): 756–61.

61. Vogt AM, Geyer H, Jahn L, et al. [Cardiomyopathy associated with uncontrolled self medication of anabolic steroids]. Z Kardiol 2002;91(4):357–62.

62. Ferenchick GS. Association of steroid abuse with cardiomyopathy in athletes. Am J Med 1991; 91(5):562.

63. Schollert PV, Bendixen PM. [Dilated cardiomyopathy in a user of anabolic steroids]. Ugeskr Laeger 1993;155(16):1217–8.

64. Ahlgrim C, Guglin M. Anabolics and cardiomyopathy in a bodybuilder: case report and literature review. J Card Fail 2009;15(6):496–500.

65. Bispo M, Valente A, Maldonado R, et al. Anabolic steroid-induced cardiomyopathy underlying acute liver failure in a young bodybuilder. World J Gastroenterol 2009;15(23):2920–2.

66. Halvorsen S, Thorsby PM, Haug E. [Acute myocardial infarction in a young man who had been using androgenic anabolic steroids]. Tidsskr Nor Laegeforen 2004;124(2):170–2.

67. Fineschi V, Baroldi G, Monciotti F, et al. Anabolic steroid abuse and cardiac sudden death: a pathologic study. Arch Pathol Lab Med 2001;125(2): 253–5.

68. Godon P, Bonnefoy E, Guerard S, et al. [Myocardial infarction and anabolic steroid use. A case report]. Arch Mal Coeur Vaiss 2000;93(7):879–83.

69. Varriale P, Mirzai-tehrane M, Sedighi A. Acute myocardial infarction associated with anabolic steroids in a young HIV-infected patient. Pharmacotherapy 1999;19(7):881–4.

70. Fisher M, Appleby M, Rittoo D, et al. Myocardial infarction with extensive intracoronary thrombus induced by anabolic steroids. Br J Clin Pract 1996;50(4):222–3.

71. Kennedy C. Myocardial infarction in association with misuse of anabolic steroids. Ulster Med J 1993;62(2):174–6.

72. Kennedy MC, Lawrence C. Anabolic steroid abuse and cardiac death. Med J Aust 1993;158(5):346–8.

73. Ferenchick GS, Adelman S. Myocardial infarction associated with anabolic steroid use in a previously healthy 37-year-old weight lifter. Am Heart J 1992; 124(2):507–8.

74. McNutt RA, Ferenchick GS, Kirlin PC, et al. Acute myocardial infarction in a 22-year-old world class weight lifter using anabolic steroids. Am J Cardiol 1988;62(1):164.

75. Huie MJ. An acute myocardial infarction occurring in an anabolic steroid user. Med Sci Sports Exerc 1994;26(4):408–13.

76. Appleby M, Fisher M, Martin M. Myocardial infarction, hyperkalaemia and ventricular tachycardia in a young male body-builder. Int J Cardiol 1994; 44(2):171–4.

77. Stergiopoulos K, Brennan JJ, Mathews R, et al. Anabolic steroids, acute myocardial infarction and polycythemia: a case report and review of the literature. Vasc Health Risk Manag 2008;4(6):1475–80.

78. Lisiewicz J, Fijalkowski P, Sankowski J. [Ischemic cerebral stroke and anabolic steroids (case report)]. Neurol Neurochir Pol 1999;32(Suppl 6): 137–9.

79. Shimada Y, Yoritaka A, Tanaka Y, et al. Cerebral infarction in a young man using high-dose anabolic steroids. J Stroke Cerebrovasc Dis 2012;21(8):906. e9-11.

80. Kennedy MC, Corrigan AB, Pilbeam ST. Myocardial infarction and cerebral haemorrhage in a young body builder taking anabolic steroids. Aust N Z J Med 1993;23(6):713.

81. Lau DH, Stiles MK, John B, et al. Atrial fibrillation and anabolic steroid abuse. Int J Cardiol 2007; 117(2):e86–7.

82. Furlanello F, Bentivegna S, Cappato R, et al. Arrhythmogenic effects of illicit drugs in athletes. Ital Heart J 2003;4(12):829–37.

83. Mewis C, Spyridopoulos I, Kuhlkamp V, et al. Manifestation of severe coronary heart disease after anabolic drug abuse. Clin Cardiol 1996;19(2): 153–5.

84. Sullivan ML, Martinez CM, Gallagher EJ. Atrial fibrillation and anabolic steroids. J Emerg Med 1999;17(5):851–7.

85. Tischer KH, Heyny-von Haussen R, Mall G, et al. [Coronary thrombosis and ectasia of coronary arteries after long-term use of anabolic steroids]. Z Kardiol 2003;92(4):326–31.

86. Ment J, Ludman PF. Coronary thrombus in a 23 year old anabolic steroid user. Heart 2002;88(4):342.

87. McCarthy K, Tang AT, Dalrymple-Hay MJ, et al. Ventricular thrombosis and systemic embolism in bodybuilders: etiology and management. Ann Thorac Surg 2000;70(2):658–60.

88. Ferenchick GS. Anabolic/androgenic steroid abuse and thrombosis: is there a connection? Med Hypotheses 1991;35(1):27–31.

89. Ferenchick G, Schwartz D, Ball M, et al. Androgenic-anabolic steroid abuse and platelet aggregation: a pilot study in weight lifters. Am J Med Sci 1992;303(2):78–82.

90. Far HR, Agren G, Thiblin I. Cardiac hypertrophy in deceased users of anabolic androgenic steroids: an investigation of autopsy findings. Cardiovasc Pathol 2012;21(4):312–6.

91. Montisci M, El Mazloum R, Cecchetto G, et al. Anabolic androgenic steroids abuse and cardiac death in athletes: morphological and toxicological findings in four fatal cases. Forensic Sci Int 2012;217(1–3):e13–8.

92. Krieg A, Scharhag J, Albers T, et al. Cardiac tissue Doppler in steroid users. Int J Sports Med 2007;28(8):638–43.

93. Montisci R, Cecchetto G, Ruscazio M, et al. Early myocardial dysfunction after chronic use of anabolic androgenic steroids: combined pulsed-wave tissue Doppler imaging and ultrasonic integrated backscatter cyclic variations analysis. J Am Soc Echocardiogr 2010;23(5):516–22.

94. Baggish AL, Weiner RB, Kanayama G, et al. Long-term anabolic-androgenic steroid use is associated with left ventricular dysfunction. Circ Heart Fail 2010;3(4):472–6.

95. Hassan NA, Salem MF, Sayed MA. Doping and effects of anabolic androgenic steroids on the heart: histological, ultrastructural, and echocardiographic assessment in strength athletes. Hum Exp Toxicol 2009;28(5):273–83.

96. D'Andrea A, Caso P, Salerno G, et al. Left ventricular early myocardial dysfunction after chronic misuse of anabolic androgenic steroids: a Doppler myocardial and strain imaging analysis. Br J Sports Med 2007;41(3):149–55.

97. Nottin S, Nguyen LD, Terbah M, et al. Cardiovascular effects of androgenic anabolic steroids in male bodybuilders determined by tissue Doppler imaging. Am J Cardiol 2006;97(6):912–5.

98. Kasikcioglu E, Oflaz H, Umman B, et al. Androgenic anabolic steroids also impair right ventricular function. Int J Cardiol 2009;134(1):123–5.

99. Nyberg F, Hallberg M. Interactions between opioids and anabolic androgenic steroids: implications for the development of addictive behavior. Int Rev Neurobiol 2012;102:189–206.

100. Luijkx T, Velthuis BK, Backx FJ, et al. Anabolic androgenic steroid use is associated with ventricular dysfunction on cardiac MRI in strength trained athletes. Int J Cardiol 2013;167(3):664–8.

101. Hartgens F, Rietjens G, Keizer HA, et al. Effects of androgenic-anabolic steroids on apolipoproteins and lipoprotein (a). Br J Sports Med 2004;38(3):253–9.

102. Thompson PD, Cullinane EM, Sady SP, et al. Contrasting effects of testosterone and stanozolol on serum lipoprotein levels. JAMA 1989;261(8):1165–8.

103. Fontana K, Oliveira HC, Leonardo MB, et al. Adverse effect of the anabolic-androgenic steroid mesterolone on cardiac remodelling and lipoprotein profile is attenuated by aerobicz exercise training. Int J Exp Pathol 2008;89(5):358–66.

104. Santora LJ, Marin J, Vangrow J, et al. Coronary calcification in body builders using anabolic steroids. Prev Cardiol 2006;9(4):198–201.

105. Smit DL, Grefhorst A, Buijs MM, et al. Prospective study on blood pressure, lipid metabolism and erythrocytosis during and after androgen abuse. Andrologia 2022;54:e14372.

106. Baggish AL, Weiner RB, Kanayama G, et al. Cardiovascular Toxicity of Illicit Anabolic-Androgenic Steroid Use. Circulation 2017;135(21):1991–2002.

107. Kanayama G, Pope HG Jr. Illicit use of androgens and other hormones: recent advances. Curr Opin Endocrinol Diabetes Obes 2012;19(3):211–9.

108. Dodge T, Hoagland MF. The use of anabolic androgenic steroids and polypharmacy: a review of the literature. Drug Alcohol Depend 2011;114(2–3):100–9.

109. Velazquez I, Alter BP. Androgens and liver tumors: Fanconi's anemia and non-Fanconi's conditions. Am J Hematol 2004;77(3):257–67.

110. Carrasco D, Prieto M, Pallardo L, et al. Multiple hepatic adenomas after long-term therapy with testosterone enanthate. Review of the literature. J Hepatol 1985;1(6):573–8.

111. Modlinski R, Fields KB. The effect of anabolic steroids on the gastrointestinal system, kidneys, and adrenal glands. Curr Sports Med Rep 2006;5(2):104–9.

112. Neri M, Bello S, Bonsignore A, et al. Anabolic androgenic steroids abuse and liver toxicity. Mini Rev Med Chem 2011;11(5):430–7.

113. Westaby D, Ogle SJ, Paradinas FJ, et al. Liver damage from long-term methyltestosterone. Lancet 1977;2(8032):262–3.

114. Karasawa T, Shikata T, Smith RD. Peliosis hepatis. Report of nine cases. Acta Pathol Jpn 1979;29(3): 457–69.

115. Schumacher J, Muller G, Klotz KF. Large hepatic hematoma and intraabdominal hemorrhage associated with abuse of anabolic steroids. New Engl J Med 1999;340(14):1123–4.

116. Daneshmend TK, Bradfield JW. Hepatic angiosarcoma associated with androgenic-anabolic steroids. Lancet 1979;2(8154):1249.

117. Falk H, Thomas LB, Popper H, et al. Hepatic angiosarcoma associated with androgenic-anabolic steroids. Lancet 1979;2(8152):1120–3.

118. Bagia S, Hewitt PM, Morris DL. Anabolic steroid-induced hepatic adenomas with spontaneous haemorrhage in a bodybuilder. Aust N Z J Surg 2000; 70(9):686–7.

119. Nakao A, Sakagami K, Nakata Y, et al. Multiple hepatic adenomas caused by long-term administration of androgenic steroids for aplastic anemia in association with familial adenomatous polyposis. J Gastroenterol 2000;35(7):557–62.

120. Gorayski P, Thompson CH, Subhash HS, et al. Hepatocellular carcinoma associated with recreational anabolic steroid use. Br J Sports Med 2008;42(1):74–5 [discussion: 75].

121. Dickerman RD, Pertusi RM, Zachariah NY, et al. Anabolic steroid-induced hepatotoxicity: is it overstated? Clin J Sport Med 1999;9(1):34–9.

122. Bachman E, Travison TG, Basaria S, et al. Testosterone induces erythrocytosis via increased erythropoietin and suppressed hepcidin: evidence for a new erythropoietin/hemoglobin set point. journals Gerontol Ser A, Biol Sci Med Sci 2014;69(6): 725–35.

123. Bachman E, Feng R, Travison T, et al. Testosterone suppresses hepcidin in men: a potential mechanism for testosterone-induced erythrocytosis. J Clin Endocrinol Metab 2010;95(10):4743–7.

124. Guo W, Bachman E, Li M, et al. Testosterone administration inhibits hepcidin transcription and is associated with increased iron incorporation into red blood cells. Aging Cell 2013;12(2):280–91.

125. Coviello AD, Kaplan B, Lakshman KM, et al. Effects of graded doses of testosterone on erythropoiesis in healthy young and older men. J Clin Endocrinol Metab 2008;93(3):914–9.

126. Palacios A, Campfield LA, McClure RD, et al. Effect of testosterone enanthate on hematopoiesis in normal men. Fertil sterility 1983;40(1):100–4.

127. Maggio M, Snyder PJ, Ceda GP, et al. Is the haematopoietic effect of testosterone mediated by erythropoietin? The results of a clinical trial in older men. Andrology 2013;1(1):24–8.

128. Ohlander SJ, Varghese B, Pastuszak AW. Erythrocytosis Following Testosterone Therapy. Sex Med Rev 2018;6(1):77–85.

129. Bhasin S, Woodhouse L, Casaburi R, et al. Older men are as responsive as young men to the anabolic effects of graded doses of testosterone on the skeletal muscle. J Clin Endocrinol Metab 2005;90(2):678–88.

130. Calof OM, Singh AB, Lee ML, et al. Adverse events associated with testosterone replacement in middle-aged and older men: a meta-analysis of randomized, placebo-controlled trials. journals Gerontol Ser A, Biol Sci Med Sci 2005;60(11): 1451–7.

131. Dobs AS, Meikle AW, Arver S, et al. Pharmacokinetics, efficacy, and safety of a permeation-enhanced testosterone transdermal system in comparison with bi-weekly injections of testosterone enanthate for the treatment of hypogonadal men. J Clin Endocrinol Metab 1999;84(10):3469–78.

132. Amory JK, Watts NB, Easley KA, et al. Exogenous testosterone or testosterone with finasteride increases bone mineral density in older men with low serum testosterone. J Clin Endocrinol Metab 2004;89(2):503–10.

133. Booij J, Kuypers J. The haemopoietic effect of nandrolone-phenylpropionate (Durabolin). Acta Physiol Pharmacol Neerl 1962;11:12–9.

134. Everse JW. [Testosterone, anabolic agents and erythropoiesis]. Hormoon 1962;26:1–11.

135. Gagnon DR, Zhang TJ, Brand FN, et al. Hematocrit and the risk of cardiovascular disease–the Framingham study: a 34-year follow-up. Am Heart J 1994;127(3):674–82.

136. Kiyohara Y, Ueda K, Hasuo Y, et al. Hematocrit as a risk factor of cerebral infarction: long-term prospective population survey in a Japanese rural community. Stroke 1986;17(4):687–92.

137. Niazi GA, Awada A, al Rajeh S, et al. Hematological values and their assessment as risk factor in Saudi patients with stroke. Acta Neurol Scand 1994; 89(6):439–45.

138. Tohgi H, Yamanouchi H, Murakami M, et al. Importance of the hematocrit as a risk factor in cerebral infarction. Stroke 1978;9(4):369–74.

139. Spiess BD, Ley C, Body SC, et al. Hematocrit value on intensive care unit entry influences the frequency of Q-wave myocardial infarction after coronary artery bypass grafting. The Institutions of the Multicenter Study of Perioperative Ischemia (McSPI) Research Group. J Thorac Cardiovasc Surg 1998;116(3):460–7.

140. Goubali A, Voukiklaris G, Kritsikis S, et al. Relation of hematocrit values to coronary heart disease, arterial hypertension, and respiratory impairment in occupational and population groups of the Athens area. Angiology 1995;46(8):719–25.

141. Burch GE, Depasquale NP. The hematocrit in patients with myocardial infarction. JAMA 1962;180: 62–3.

142. Sorlie PD, Garcia-Palmieri MR, Costas R Jr, et al. Hematocrit and risk of coronary heart disease: the Puerto Rico Health Program. Am Heart J 1981;101(4):456–61.

143. Carter C, McGee D, Reed D, et al. Hematocrit and the risk of coronary heart disease: the Honolulu Heart Program. Am Heart J 1983;105(4): 674–9.

144. Horn S, Gregory P, Guskiewicz KM. Self-reported anabolic-androgenic steroids use and musculoskeletal injuries: findings from the center for the study of retired athletes health survey of retired NFL players. Am J Phys Med Rehabil 2009;88(3): 192–200.

145. Laseter JT, Russell JA. Anabolic steroid-induced tendon pathology: a review of the literature. Med Sci Sports Exerc 1991;23(1):1–3.

146. Pertusi R, Dickerman RD, McConathy WJ. Evaluation of aminotransferase elevations in a bodybuilder using anabolic steroids: hepatitis or rhabdomyolysis? J Am Osteopath Assoc 2001; 101(7):391–4.

147. Adamson R, Rambaran C, D'Cruz DP. Anabolic steroid-induced rhabdomyolysis. Hosp Med 2005; 66(6):362.

148. Evans NA, Bowrey DJ, Newman GR. Ultrastructural analysis of ruptured tendon from anabolic steroid users. Injury 1998;29(10):769–73.

149. Wood TO, Cooke PH, Goodship AE. The effect of exercise and anabolic steroids on the mechanical properties and crimp morphology of the rat tendon. Am J Sports Med 1988;16(2):153–8.

150. Inhofe PD, Grana WA, Egle D, et al. The effects of anabolic steroids on rat tendon. An ultrastructural, biomechanical, and biochemical analysis. Am J Sports Med 1995;23(2):227–32.

151. Scott MJ 3rd, Scott AM. Effects of anabolic-androgenic steroids on the pilosebaceous unit. Cutis 1992;50(2):113–6.

152. Winnett G, Cranfield L, Almond M. Apparent renal disease due to elevated creatinine levels associated with the use of boldenone. Nephrol Dial Transplant 2011;26(2):744–7.

153. Herlitz LC, Markowitz GS, Farris AB, et al. Development of focal segmental glomerulosclerosis after anabolic steroid abuse. J Am Soc Nephrol 2010; 21(1):163–72.

154. Crampin AC, Lamagni TL, Hope VD, et al. The risk of infection with HIV and hepatitis B in individuals who inject steroids in England and Wales. Epidemiol Infect 1998;121(2):381–6.

155. Centers for Disease C, Prevention. Methicillin-resistant staphylococcus aureus infections among competitive sports participants–Colorado, Indiana, Pennsylvania, and Los Angeles County, 2000-2003. MMWR Morb Mortal Wkly Rep 2003;52(33): 793–5.

156. Bolding G, Sherr L, Maguire M, et al. HIV risk behaviours among gay men who use anabolic steroids. Addiction 1999;94(12):1829–35.

157. Pope HG Jr, Kouri EM, Powell KF, et al. Anabolic-androgenic steroid use among 133 prisoners. Compr Psychiatry 1996;37(5):322–7.

158. Klotz F, Petersson A, Hoffman O, et al. The significance of anabolic androgenic steroids in a Swedish prison population. Compr Psychiatry 2010; 51(3):312–8.

159. Lundholm L, Kall K, Wallin S, et al. Use of anabolic androgenic steroids in substance abusers arrested for crime. Drug Alcohol Depend 2010;111(3): 222–6.

160. Tan RS, Vasudevan D. Use of clomiphene citrate to reverse premature andropause secondary to steroid abuse. Fertil sterility 2003;79(1):203–5.

161. Guay AT, Jacobson J, Perez JB, et al. Clomiphene increases free testosterone levels in men with both secondary hypogonadism and erectile dysfunction: who does and does not benefit? Int J impotence Res 2003;15(3):156–65.

162. Habous M, Giona S, Tealab A, et al. Clomiphene citrate and human chorionic gonadotropin are both effective in restoring testosterone in hypogonadism: a short-course randomized study. BJU Int 2018;122(5):889–97.

163. Moskovic DJ, Katz DJ, Akhavan A, et al. Clomiphene citrate is safe and effective for long-term management of hypogonadism. BJU Int 2012; 110(10):1524–8.

164. Katz DJ, Nabulsi O, Tal R, et al. Outcomes of clomiphene citrate treatment in young hypogonadal men. BJU Int 2012;110(4):573–8.

165. Politou M, Gialeraki A, Merkouri E, et al. Central retinal vein occlusion secondary to clomiphene treatment in a male carrier of factor V Leiden. Genet Test Mol Biomarkers 2009;13(2):155–7.

166. Zahid M, Arshad A, Zafar A, et al. Intracranial venous thrombosis in a man taking clomiphene citrate. BMJ Case Rep 2016;2016. bcr2016217403.

167. Finkel DM, Phillips JL, Snyder PJ. Stimulation of spermatogenesis by gonadotropins in men with hypogonadotropic hypogonadism. New Engl J Med 1985;313(11):651–5.

168. Bhasin S, Brito JP, Cunningham GR, et al. Testosterone Therapy in Men With Hypogonadism: An Endocrine Society Clinical Practice Guideline. J Clin Endocrinol Metab 2018;103(5):1715–44.

169. Shin YS, Park JK. The Optimal Indication for Testosterone Replacement Therapy in Late Onset Hypogonadism. J Clin Med 2019;8(2):209.

170. Corona G, Krausz C. Late-onset hypogonadism a challenging task for the andrology field. Andrology 2020;8(6):1504–5.

171. Snyder P. Testosterone treatment of late-onset hypogonadism - benefits and risks. Rev Endocr

Metab Disord 2022. https://doi.org/10.1007/s11154-022-09712-1.

172. Hershberger LG, Shipley EG, Meyer RK. Myotrophic activity of 19-nortestosterone and other steroids determined by modified levator ani muscle method. Proc Soc Exp Biol Med 1953;83(1):175–80.

173. Kicman AT. Pharmacology of anabolic steroids. Br J Pharmacol 2008;154(3):502–21.

174. Kuhn CM. Anabolic steroids. Recent Prog Horm Res 2002;57:411–34.

175. Reeves PT, Herndon DN, Tanksley JD, et al. Five-Year Outcomes after Long-Term Oxandrolone Administration in Severely Burned Children: A Randomized Clinical Trial. Shock 2016;45(4):367–74.

176. Li H, Guo Y, Yang Z, et al. The efficacy and safety of oxandrolone treatment for patients with severe burns: A systematic review and meta-analysis. Burns 2016;42(4):717–27.

177. Mulligan K, Schambelan M. Anabolic treatment with GH, IGF-I, or anabolic steroids in patients with HIV-associated wasting. Int J Cardiol 2002;85(1):151–9.

178. Berger JR, Pall L, Hall CD, et al. Oxandrolone in AIDS-wasting myopathy. AIDS 1996;10(14):1657–62.

179. Hengge UR, Stocks K, Faulkner S, et al. Oxymetholone for the treatment of HIV-wasting: a double-blind, randomized, placebo-controlled phase III trial in eugonadal men and women. HIV Clin Trials 2003;4(3):150–63.

180. Gold J, Batterham MJ, Rekers H, et al. Effects of nandrolone decanoate compared with placebo or testosterone on HIV-associated wasting. HIV Med 2006;7(3):146–55.

181. Chen CT, Lin SH, Chen JS, et al. Muscle wasting in hemodialysis patients: new therapeutic strategies for resolving an old problem. ScientificWorldJournal 2013;2013:643954.

182. Fenichel GM, Griggs RC, Kissel J, et al. A randomized efficacy and safety trial of oxandrolone in the treatment of Duchenne dystrophy. Neurology 2001;56(8):1075–9.

183. Wood CL, Page J, Foggin J, et al. The impact of testosterone therapy on quality of life in adolescents with Duchenne muscular dystrophy. Neuromuscul Disord 2021;31(12):1259–65.

184. Lee SL, Lim A, Munns C, et al. Effect of Testosterone Treatment for Delayed Puberty in Duchenne Muscular Dystrophy. Horm Res Paediatr 2020;93(2):108–18.

185. Rosenfeld J, King RM, Smith JE. Oxandrolone in ALS: preliminary analysis. Amyotroph Lateral Scler Other Mot Neuron Disord 2000;1(Suppl 4):21–5 [discussion: 25–6].

186. Sharma S, Arneja A, McLean L, et al. Anabolic steroids in COPD: a review and preliminary results of a randomized trial. Chron Respir Dis 2008;5(3):169–76.

187. Yeh SS, DeGuzman B, Kramer T, et al. Reversal of COPD-associated weight loss using the anabolic agent oxandrolone. Chest 2002;122(2):421–8.

188. Svartberg J. Androgens and chronic obstructive pulmonary disease. Curr Opin Endocrinol Diabetes Obes 2010;17(3):257–61.

189. Baillargeon J, Urban RJ, Zhang W, et al. Testosterone replacement therapy and hospitalization rates in men with COPD. Chron Respir Dis 2019;16. 1479972318793004.

190. Orr R, Fiatarone Singh M. The anabolic androgenic steroid oxandrolone in the treatment of wasting and catabolic disorders: review of efficacy and safety. Drugs 2004;64(7):725–50.

191. Krug K. [Pathophysiology of aplastic anemia and its treatment with methenolone enanthate]. Z Gesamte Inn Med 1980;35(22):809–12.

192. Doney K, Storb R, Buckner CD, et al. Treatment of aplastic anemia with antithymocyte globulin, high-dose corticosteroids, and androgens. Exp Hematol 1987;15(3):239–42.

193. Shahani S, Braga-Basaria M, Maggio M, et al. Androgens and erythropoiesis: past and present. J endocrinological Invest 2009;32(8):704–16.

194. Duarte L, Lopez Sandoval R, Esquivel F, et al. Androstane therapy of aplastic anaemia. Acta Haematol 1972;47(3):140–5.

195. Palva IP, Wasastjerna C. Treatment of aplastic anaemia with methenolone. Acta Haematol 1972;47(1):13–20.

196. Sacks P, Gale D, Bothwell TH, et al. Oxymetholone therapy in aplastic and other refractory anaemias. S Afr Med J 1972;46(43):1607–15.

197. Navarro JF, Mora C, Macia M, et al. Randomized prospective comparison between erythropoietin and androgens in CAPD patients. Kidney Int 2002;61(4):1537–44.

198. Gaughan WJ, Liss KA, Dunn SR, et al. A 6-month study of low-dose recombinant human erythropoietin alone and in combination with androgens for the treatment of anemia in chronic hemodialysis patients. Am J Kidney Dis 1997;30(4):495–500.

199. Teruel JL, Aguilera A, Marcen R, et al. Androgen therapy for anaemia of chronic renal failure. Indications in the erythropoietin era. Scand J Urol Nephrol 1996;30(5):403–8.

200. Mirand EA, Murphy GP, Steeves RA, et al. Erythropoietin activity in anephric, allotransplanted, unilaterally nephrectomized and intact man. J Lab Clin Med 1969;73(1):121–8.

201. DeGowin RL, Lavender AR, Forland M, et al. Erythropoiesis and erythropoietin in patients with chronic renal failure treated with hemodialysis and testosterone. Ann Intern Med 1970;72(6):913–8.

202. Richardson JR Jr, Weinstein MB. Erythropoietic response of dialyzed patients to testosterone administration. Ann Intern Med 1970;73(3):403–7.

203. Soufir JC, Meduri G, Ziyyat A. Spermatogenetic inhibition in men taking a combination of oral medroxyprogesterone acetate and percutaneous testosterone as a male contraceptive method. Hum Reprod 2011;26(7):1708–14.

204. Contraceptive efficacy of testosterone-induced azoospermia in normal men. World Health Organization Task Force on methods for the regulation of male fertility. Lancet 1990;336(8721):955–9.

205. World Health Organization Task Force on Methods for the Regulation of Male F. Contraceptive efficacy of testosterone-induced azoospermia and oligozoospermia in normal men. Fertil sterility 1996; 65(4):821–9.

206. Turner L, Conway AJ, Jimenez M, et al. Contraceptive efficacy of a depot progestin and androgen combination in men. J Clin Endocrinol Metab 2003;88(10):4659–67.

207. Gu YQ, Wang XH, Xu D, et al. A multicenter contraceptive efficacy study of injectable testosterone undecanoate in healthy Chinese men. J Clin Endocrinol Metab 2003;88(2):562–8.

208. Gu Y, Liang X, Wu W, et al. Multicenter contraceptive efficacy trial of injectable testosterone undecanoate in Chinese men. J Clin Endocrinol Metab 2009;94(6):1910–5.

209. Thirumalai A, Ceponis J, Amory JK, et al. Effects of 28 Days of Oral Dimethandrolone Undecanoate in Healthy Men: A Prototype Male Pill. J Clin Endocrinol Metab 2019;104(2):423–32.

210. Yuen F, Thirumalai A, Pham C, et al. Daily Oral Administration of the Novel Androgen 11beta-MNTDC Markedly Suppresses Serum Gonadotropins in Healthy Men. J Clin Endocrinol Metab 2020;105(3):e835–47.

211. Anawalt BD, Roth MY, Ceponis J, et al. Combined nestorone-testosterone gel suppresses serum gonadotropins to concentrations associated with effective hormonal contraception in men. Andrology 2019;7(6):878–87.

212. Ip EJ, Barnett MJ, Tenerowicz MJ, et al. Women and anabolic steroids: an analysis of a dozen users. Clin J Sport Med 2010;20(6):475–81.

213. Gruber AJ, Pope HG Jr. Psychiatric and medical effects of anabolic-androgenic steroid use in women. Psychother Psychosom 2000;69(1):19–26.

Testosterone Assays

Brendan King, MD, Caleb Natale, MD, Wayne J.G. Hellstrom, MD*

KEYWORDS

• Testosterone assays • Hypogonadism • Total testosterone • Free testosterone

KEY POINTS

- Accurate and precise measurement of testosterone is necessary to diagnose and manage hypogonadism in men as well as other endocrine conditions.
- Measurement of free testosterone and the bioavailable fraction may be clinically useful in some patient populations and clinical scenarios, particularly in men with borderline low total testosterone.
- Mass spectrometry is the gold standard measurement modality for total testosterone but is not available in many standard clinical laboratories due to barriers related to cost and technical challenges.
- Testosterone measurements should be performed in the morning in a fasting state with any low serum testosterone measurements performed in duplicate.

The accurate detection and quantification of serum testosterone levels is necessary for the diagnosis of hypogonadism in men, evaluation of endocrine abnormalities, and monitoring and titration of testosterone therapy, among other clinical scenarios. Achieving accurate and precise measurements is accompanied by a host of challenges such as deficiencies in standardization across laboratories, variability in reference ranges, expenses related to gold standard equipment, and technical as well as logistical challenges in performing these assays. Total testosterone levels include testosterone that is specifically bound to sex hormone-binding globulin (SHBG), nonspecifically bound to albumin, corticosteroid-binding globulin, and orosomucoid, as well as a small percentage of unbound hormone within the serum. According to the free hormone hypothesis, the unbound fraction of testosterone represents the biologically active component of total testosterone, although this theory is debated. Other evidence suggests that the bioavailable fraction, which refers to free testosterone plus nonspecifically bound testosterone, is a better indicator of biological activity than the free testosterone. Measurement of total testosterone remains the most accessible for standard laboratories and can be accomplished by a variety of measures, which include immunoassays (IAs), which are relatively inexpensive, rapid, and technically facile; and mass spectrometry (MS), which is the gold standard but is associated with higher technological costs and is more technically challenging and time consuming. The measurement of free testosterone can be accomplished by equilibrium dialysis, IAs, and calculations that use algorithms to estimate the value based on measurements of total testosterone, SHBG, and albumin within the sample of interest. Equilibrium dialysis is the gold standard, which requires standardized conditions and is therefore more technically challenging and time consuming than the other methods. IAs are highly inaccurate and, although widely available and inexpensive, are not recommended. Bioavailable testosterone can be estimated via precipitation of SHBG-bound testosterone followed by assay of tracer-labeled testosterone and calculation. Reference ranges vary among society's guidelines, but the lower limit of normal testosterone in men is set at greater than 230 ng/dL by all major societies surveyed for this article. Efforts to adapt reference ranges to different populations, including age-adjusted populations, have augmented our understanding of normal testosterone levels in men. Further

Department of Urology, Tulane University School of Medicine, #8642 1430 Tulane Avenue, New Orleans, LA 70112, USA
* Corresponding author.
E-mail address: whellst@tulane.edu

Urol Clin N Am 49 (2022) 665–677
https://doi.org/10.1016/j.ucl.2022.07.009
0094-0143/22/© 2022 Elsevier Inc. All rights reserved.

collaboration aimed at establishing common reference ranges, as well as standardizing varied commercial products, is necessary to systematize the interpretation of testosterone assays, the diagnosis, and the monitoring of hypogonadism, as well as other endocrine conditions (**Box 1**).

INTRODUCTION

Testosterone is the primary androgenic hormone in humans.[1] The accurate detection and quantification of serum testosterone levels is an increasingly necessary component of standard clinical care for practicing urologists as well as for general practice medical providers.

Testosterone replacement therapy (TRT) as treatment of testosterone deficiency (TD), transgender health care, and endocrine abnormalities, among other clinical scenarios, requires precise and accurate detection of serum testosterone.

An accurate diagnosis of male hypogonadism depends on the reliable quantification of serum testosterone levels. In the case of TRT, clinical consensus guidelines consistently recommend that only men meeting criteria for TD should be treated.[2] Importantly, low testosterone alone does not define TD. Rather, a diagnosis of TD must include the presence of symptoms and/or signs associated with low testosterone in addition to documented low serum total testosterone levels.[3] To diagnose hypogonadism, the American Urological Association (AUA) requires symptoms and/or signs such as fatigue, cognitive dysfunction, loss of body hair, and depressed mood, as well as by total testosterone 300 ng/dL (10.4 nmol/L).[3] Furthermore, all patients receiving testosterone therapy require careful laboratory monitoring for safety and efficacy as well as to ensure that testosterone levels are titrated to target levels. A variety of laboratory assays and protocols exist to measure testosterone. Measurement by testosterone assays is a critical component of diagnosing hypogonadism in men, in addition to other endocrine conditions. Assay technologies, protocols, and target ranges can vary by the clinical or commercial laboratory running the samples. Recommended diagnostic and therapeutic ranges are also not standardized.

Challenges to obtaining accurate assays of serum testosterone include diurnal fluctuations in serum testosterone, a wide range of normal values of testosterone, and technical as well as logistical challenges in performing assays. In this article, we seek to elucidate the variety of testosterone assays available and the manner in which these assays are interpreted.

THE AVAILABILITY OF TESTOSTERONE IN THE SERUM AND THE FREE HORMONE HYPOTHESIS

Total testosterone refers to the sum of primary androgenic hormones circulating within the serum. Total testosterone levels include testosterone bound specifically to SHBG, testosterone bound nonspecifically to albumin, corticosteroid-binding globulin, and orosomucoid, and a small percentage of unbound hormone in the serum[4,5] (**Fig. 1**). The term *free testosterone* refers to this small unbound fraction. The term *bioavailable fraction* refers to the free testosterone as well as the nonspecifically bound testosterone. Measurement of the fraction of hormone that is available at the cellular level in target tissues, even in ideal laboratory settings, is currently limited to the estimation of the bioavailable fraction.

The *free hormone hypothesis* states that the unbound fraction of testosterone represents the biologically active component of total testosterone at target tissues.[6] The free hormone hypothesis

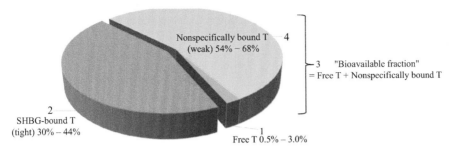

Fig. 1. The approximate fractions of testosterone circulating within the serum, including the unbound fraction (free testosterone), the nonspecifically bound fraction, and the tightly bound fraction.

continues to be highly debated.[7] Subsequent studies estimate that the bioavailable fraction more accurately represents the biologically active proportion of testosterone within the serum.[8,9] More recent evidence suggests that testosterone bound to SHBG may even exert a biological effect in certain tissues, such as in the prostate.[7,10]

Evidence from a Large Epidemiological Study

The European Male Aging Study is a multicenter, prospective cohort study examining aging-related symptoms in men, specifically focusing on the effects of age-related changes in hormone levels and their related symptoms.[11] A significant association was found between decreased libido, morning erections, and erectile dysfunction and testosterone levels of < 11 nmol/L (317 ng/dL) and free testosterone levels of < 280 pmol/L in this large-scale, population-based study.[11,12]

These threshold values indicate the likelihood of sexual symptoms occurring more significantly in men with these levels compared to men with normal values of testosterone. However, the probability of these sexual symptoms increased with decreasing levels of total testosterone and free testosterone, therefore revealing an inverse relationship. The results of this study suggest that there may be utility in measuring free testosterone for diagnostic purposes in symptomatic men with normal or borderline low total testosterone levels.

TESTOSTERONE MEASUREMENTS

Measurement of total testosterone is typically preferred in standard clinical settings due to the challenging nature of measuring free testosterone. Equilibrium dialysis methods of free testosterone quantification remain the current gold standard, but these assays are generally too complex for standard laboratories, as their performance can be affected by assay conditions that result in high assay variability.[6,7,13] In a 2017 study by Cao and colleagues,[14] in which four samples

were distributed to 142 accredited laboratories to study assay performance compared to target values determined by using the reference measurement procedures operated by the Centers for Disease Control and Prevention Clinical Reference Laboratory, significant variability in accuracy and precision between the types of assays performed and the laboratories performing the assays was reported. Cao and colleagues[14] ultimately concluded that incorrect assay calibration and insufficient analytical specificity were most likely responsible for the high variability.

Furthermore, the lack of common reference intervals, which rely on faulty models of testosterone to SHBG ratios, fosters potential misinterpretation of estimates of free testosterone.[7] Similar challenges impede the measurement of bioavailable testosterone. Available assays are technically difficult and not commonly performed in typical clinical laboratories.[7] Because of the significant interassay variability, programs such as the CDC Hormone Standardization Program (CDC HoSt) were established to accredit the performance of specific laboratories and assays.

Regarding testosterone, CDC HoSt certifies the performance of assays at distinct laboratories within the concentration range of 2.50 to 1000 ng/dL for total testosterone and designates those laboratories that meet the performance criterion of ±6.4% mean bias when compared to the CDC reference measurement procedure for total testosterone.[15] Moreover, the AUA guidelines recommend measuring total testosterone levels at the same laboratory and using the same assay on two separate occasions in an early morning fashion to ensure comparable measurements.[3]

TOTAL TESTOSTERONE
Immunoassays

IAs have been widely utilized in clinical practice, given their relative ease of use, simplicity, cost, acceptable performance at normal testosterone levels, and scalability (**Table 1**).

Table 1
A select summary of assays available to measure total testosterone

			Assays for Total Testosterone		
Assays	**Mechanisms**	**Units**	**Coefficients of Variation**	**Advantages**	**Disadvantages**
Immunoassay (including radioimmunoassay and enzyme immunoassay)	• Serum mixed with T antibodies and tracer • Tracer can be radioisotope (RIA), enzyme (EIA), fluorescent, or chemiluminescent compound	ng/dL	• Intraassay: −14% to +19% • CV most pronounced at low T values (40% in samples with TT < 100 ng/dL)	• Rapid and simple • Inexpensive • Commonly utilized • High-throughput • Reference range data available	• Significant interassay variability • Reduced accuracy at low/high T levels • Interfering factors (heterophile antibodies in serum)
Liquid chromatography-mass spectrometry	• Ionizes molecules and measures mass-to-charge ratios	ng/dL	• ±6.4% (to maintain CDC approval status)	• Gold standard • Excellent sensitivity and specificity, even at low T concentrations (<40 ng/dL) • Simultaneous measurement of multiple steroids	• Not FDA approved • Low-throughput • Labor intensive • Expensive

For these reasons, most of the total testosterone reference ranges were established by using these methods. In short, IAs rely on tracer-linked testosterone molecules that compete with native testosterone in samples for the binding of testosterone antibodies. The tracer molecule may be an enzyme (*enzyme immunoassay, EIA*), a radioisotope (*radioimmunoassay, RIA*), chemiluminescent (chemiluminescent immunoassay), or fluorescent (*fluoroimmunoassay, FIA*) compound. The disadvantages of performing IA include the technical expertise and additional time needed for testosterone extraction/chromatography as well as reduced accuracy at low or high testosterone levels. RIA are accompanied by the additional disadvantage of generating radioactive waste.[16]

Wang and colleagues evaluated the results of four common automated IA and two manual IA related to 62 eugonadal and 60 hypogonadal men. As demonstrated by Wang and colleagues,[17] who used liquid chromatography-tandem mass spectrometry (LC-MS/MS) as the gold standard, none of the six different IAs tested were of sufficient accuracy at low serum testosterone levels. Despite these findings, Wang and colleagues[17] stated that, from a clinical standpoint, several of the IAs in the study would be appropriate for use in adult males with low testosterone (100 ng/dL) levels, as these men would have been diagnosed with hypogonadism and treated accordingly. In a similar study, Taieb and colleagues[18] investigated commercially available testosterone IAs for accuracy in the measurement of serum testosterone in 50 men, 55 women, and 11 children. Compared with the gas chromatography-mass spectrometry analysis, which is considered the gold standard in this study, none of the 10 IAs tested were sufficiently reliable in women and children whose testosterone levels were low (<1.7 nmol/L, <49.05 ng/dL) or very low (0.17 nmol/L, 4.9 ng/dL).[18]

Mass Spectrometry

MS-based assays remain the gold standard for quantification of total testosterone levels. Despite higher costs, MS has become increasingly more utilized in clinical practice in part due to its higher sensitivity and specificity at both low and high testosterone levels compared to IAs, which have been shown to vary significantly, particularly at low testosterone levels.[19,20] From 2012 to 2015, nearly a fivefold increase in the use of MS-based assays was reported by the College of American Pathologists.[14]

Additional advantages of MS include the ability to measure multiple steroid levels simultaneously, simple sample preparation wherein nonderivatized steroids can be analyzed directly; high recovery with improved signal-to-noise ratio; and lower interference.[17]

In contrast to IA, MS involves the ionization of serum compounds and subsequent measurement of their mass-to-charge ratios or molecular weight. Preanalysis extraction or chromatography (gas or liquid) prior to MS can be performed to separate hormones and proteins that could otherwise affect the accurate measurement of testosterone. The MS subtype, LC-MS/MS, which couples the liquid chromatography technique of chemical separation to the MS technique, has been an increasingly adopted high-throughput and accurate testosterone assay in clinical practice and research.[19] Although considerable interlaboratory variability exists with MS, this remains a significant improvement from the variability inherent to commercially available IAs.[21] The high complexity of laboratory equipment required and the relatively high expense of running MS remain the predominant obstacles to its widespread adoption.[22]

FREE TESTOSTERONE
Equilibrium Dialysis

Equilibrium dialysis, if performed under standardized conditions, represents the gold standard for detection of free testosterone[23] (**Table 2**). This method utilizes a semipermeable membrane to isolate testosterone bound to protein by molecular weight.[24] Free testosterone, which is not bound to protein, is able to equilibrate across the semipermeable membrane due to its lower molecular weight. Testosterone present within the dialysate can then be measured via direct or indirect methods.[7] Direct methods include LC-MS/MS to measure the amount of free testosterone within the dialysate. Alternatively, free testosterone can be measured directly via an IA or indirectly via assessment with the addition of a small quantity of testosterone radiotracer.[7] Analytical performance during the measurement step highly impacts the accuracy of this measurement.

Challenges related to equilibrium dialysis include the impact of dilution of samples as well as the susceptibility of dialysis based on temperature and pH.[25] These challenges highlight the crucial maintenance of a standardized environment. The utility of equilibrium dialysis is also impacted by the time-consuming movement of dialysate across the membrane, given separation can take up to 16 hours to complete. A modified method of equilibrium dialysis, known as *ultrafiltration,* utilizes centrifugation to force the sample through the semipermeable membrane. This method reduces the time necessary for the sample

Table 2
A select summary of assays available to measure free testosterone

Assays		Mechanisms	Units	Coefficients of Variation	Advantages	Disadvantages
	Assays for Free Testosterone					
Equilibrium dialysis		• Serum placed in dialysis chamber • Tracer-labeled T added to serum • Equilibrium achieved • Low molecular weight permeable membrane restricts passage of small molecules • Proportion of bound & free-labeled T assessed	pg/dL	• Interassay: 6.8% • Intraassay: 10.0%	• Gold standard • Excellent sensitivity and specificity • Reproducible	• Time/labor-intensive • Low-throughput • Technically challenging • Expensive • Relies on accuracy of TT assay • Tracer impurities may compromise results
Calculated FT		• Law of mass action (Nanjee & Wheeler, Sodergard, Vermeulen)	pg/mL	• Interassay: 18–30%	• Simple • Rapid • Has correlated well in some series with equilibrium dialysis	• Relies on TT and SHBG assay accuracy • Accuracy relies on equilibrium dissociation constants for binding of SHBG and albumin to testosterone • High interassay variability • Tends to overestimate true value
Direct (Ultracentrifugation, Analog)		• Radiolabeled T is added to sample and allowed to reach equilibrium with T in serum • Free T is separated by centrifugal ultrafiltration • Radioactivity of protein-free ultrafiltrate is measured and used to calculate % free T	pg/mL	• Interassay: 8.9% • Intraassay: 10.3%	• Method shows promise but additional studies required to measure assay performance across the range of free T values	• Low-throughput • Technically challenging • Relies on accuracy of TT measurement

to reach equilibrium. Analytical performance has been noted to be generally comparable to standard equilibrium dialysis while requiring significantly shorter operating times.[26,27] An additional challenge with ultracentrifugation is the adsorption of samples to the ultrafiltration filter.[25] The percentage of samples lost in this manner likely varies according to the commercial filter being used.

Analogue Immunoassays

Use of commercially available IA kits for the measurement of free testosterone confers many of the same benefits as described earlier. IAs, which are widely available at large and small laboratories, are relatively inexpensive and easily performed over short operating times. Measurements of free testosterone, which is present at relatively low concentrations, are often inaccurate due to alterations in the levels of SHBG.[28] For these reasons, the use of IAs is not recommended for the measurement of free testosterone.[29]

Calculated Free Testosterone

Free testosterone can be measured indirectly via several established calculations using algorithms to estimate bioavailable testosterone, free androgen index (FAI = TT/SHBG × 100), and free testosterone index, for example. Additional examples include the Sodergard, Nanjee–Wheeler, Vermeulen, and Ly–Handelsman methods that estimate free testosterone by using measured testosterone, albumin, and SHBG concentrations.[30] Several studies have investigated the predictive accuracy of calculated free testosterone, including one by Morris and colleagues,[31] which demonstrated high predictability by using and comparing total testosterone to other tested modalities in assessing for biochemical hypogonadism. Using multiple linear regression analysis on their training cohort, Morris and colleagues derived an equation, lnBioT = −0.266 + (0.955 × lnTT)−(0.228 × lnSHBG), where ln = natural log, BioT = bioavailable testosterone, TT = total testosterone, and SHBG = sex hormone-binding globulin, and demonstrated a high correlation between derived values and true values for bioavailable testosterone.[31] Calculation of free testosterone relies on the measurement of total testosterone, SHBG, and albumin within the sample of interest. Calculation of free testosterone is performed according to the law of mass action while utilizing the specific dissociation constants of the other analytes measured within the sample. In this method, the measurement accuracy of the concentrations of analytes determines the accuracy of the calculated free testosterone value.

Multiple algorithms exist within the literature, including examples derived from equilibrium binding[4] and empirically derived examples devised from the results of computer modeling based on known concentrations of the analytes of interest.[32,33]

BIOAVAILABLE TESTOSTERONE
Ammonium Sulfate Precipitation of Sex Hormone-Binding Globulin-Bound Testosterone

As a technique used to measure bioavailable testosterone, ammonium sulfate precipitation involves the mixing of tracer-labeled testosterone with serum followed by the precipitation of SHBG via the addition of ammonium sulfate (**Table 3**). Protocols often utilize saturated ammonium sulfate solution in a 1:1 ratio with the sample specimen. The remaining tracer-labeled testosterone is then multiplied by total testosterone to yield an estimation of bioavailable testosterone in serum. Although this technique correlates well with equilibrium dialysis, it has several disadvantages such as its reliability on the accuracy of the total testosterone assay and the potential impact of tracer impurities on results.[19]

An alternative to precipitation of SHBG with ammonium sulfate has been proposed with the use of concanavalin A separation.[34] Early evidence suggests that this method may have increased specificity over ammonium sulfate.[35] Giton and colleagues compared the results of 131 samples assessed for bioavailable testosterone using both ammonium sulfate precipitation and concanavalin A separation methods. They found similar results from both methods.

Concanavalin A has the benefit of eliminating errors associated with nonspecific albumin precipitation that may occur in poorly controlled assay conditions.[35] Further evaluation of this relatively novel method should precede its adoption into clinical practice.

REFERENCE RANGES

Since a standard reference range for the distribution of circulating concentrations of testosterone in healthy men remains variable and therefore undefined, there is no consensus on the accepted lower testosterone limits. Rigorously derived reference ranges serve as the mainstay of the contemporary approach to making medical diagnoses, including hypogonadism. According to a guideline supported by the European Association of Urology, International Society of Andrology, International Society for the Study of Aging Male,

Table 3
A select summary of assays available to measure bioavailable testosterone

Assays	Mechanisms	Units	Coefficients of Variation	Advantages	Disadvantages
		Assays for Bioavailable Testosterone			
Ammonium sulfate precipitation	• Tracer-labeled T added to serum • SHBG precipitated via addition of ammonium sulfate • Remaining tracer multiplied by TT	ng/dL	• Interassay: 7.9% • Intraassay: 7.2%	• Excellent sensitivity and specificity • Correlates well with equilibrium dialysis	• Time/labor intensive • Technically challenging • Low throughput • Relies on accuracy of TT assay • Tracer impurities may compromise results

European Academy of Andrology, and the American Society of Andrology, TT levels of < 230 ng/dL (8 nmol/L) in young men would benefit from TRT, while TT > 350 ng/dL (12.1 nmol/L) does not require treatment.[36] In contrast, Endocrine Society guidelines endorse a lower TT threshold for consideration of TRT at 280 to 300 ng/dL (9.7 to 10.4 nmol/L), whereas the AUA guidelines support < 300 ng/dL (10.4 nmol/L) as a reasonable cut-off level [3291].

Given the widespread adoption of MS in clinical practice, reference ranges for testosterone concentrations in healthy men have been established to clearly define the diagnosis of androgen deficiency. For example, Bhasin and colleagues[37] described reference ranges in a cohort of 456 men (aged 19–40 years) from the Framingham Heart Study Generation 3. In this community-based sample of nonobese, healthy men without significant risk factors or comorbidities, such as diabetes mellitus, hypertension, cardiovascular disease, tobacco use, or dyslipidemia, the mean TT was 724 ng/dL (25.1 nmol/L). The upper (97.5%) and lower (2.5%) intervals were 1197 ng/dL (41.5 nmol/L) and 348 ng/dL (12.1 nmol/L), respectively.[37]

Similar data have been published in other populations.

Age-Specific Reference Ranges

Male testosterone levels have been demonstrated to decrease with age. Originally a controversial conclusion, the decrease in bioavailable testosterone in aging men compared to their 40-year-old counterparts has been shown in a large series of cross-sectional and longitudinal studies.[38] The natural decline in TT levels with age and the lack of defined, age-specific thresholds for distinct symptom complexes add to the challenge of establishing reference ranges.[39]

For example, in a 2012 study that included 3690 elderly, community-dwelling men (>70 years, mean age 77 years), Yeap and colleagues[39] reported a mean TT of 378 ng/dL (13.1 nmol/L) with upper (97.5%) and lower (2.5%) reference ranges of 693 ng/dL (24 nmol/L) and 145 ng/dL (5 nmol/L), respectively. More specifically, in a subset of the study population that included 394 men (aged 76.1 years ± 3.2 years) who described themselves as in excellent or very good health, without cancer, cardiovascular disease, depression, dementia, or diabetes, and with no history of smoking, the mean as well as the upper and lower reference ranges were similar to the entire cohort.[39] In this reference group, the mean, 97.5%, and 2.5% TT levels were 406 ng/dL (14.1 nmol/L), 739 ng/dL (25.6 nmol/L), and 184 ng/dL (6.4 nmol/L),

respectively.[39] Using these reported cutoffs for the entire cohort of 3690 men, those with hypogonadism, defined as below the 2.5% reference range, had increased odds of diabetes, frailty, and cardiovascular disease.[39] The men categorized as hypogonadal in this sample population also had a higher odds ratio for these outcomes.[39]

As evidenced by Yeap and colleagues and other researchers, application of one reference range to all age groups may overestimate the prevalence of low testosterone in elderly populations compared with a standard group within the corresponding age bracket. Furthermore, laboratory reference ranges are not standardized to consider age-related testosterone standards.[40] While some laboratories may apply age-related standards, others may not. Age-related discrepancies are further complicated by the fact that while serum testosterone levels decline with age, there is an age-associated increase in SHBG of about 1.3–1.6% per year.[41] This can further exacerbate the decrease in bioavailable testosterone in aging men.[38] In the population-based Massachusetts Male Aging Study, bioavailable testosterone decreased by 2–3% per year.

Standardization of Reference Ranges

The distribution of testosterone levels has been shown to vary across populations of men from different geographic regions. In addition to biological or environmental factors, interassay and interlaboratory differences also contribute to these reported variations in reference ranges.[42] It is unclear whether reported reference ranges from one study population can be applied more broadly to other populations of men from different parts of the world. Additionally, certain disease processes and therapeutics can alter testosterone levels and further complicate the applicability of reference ranges. Diabetes mellitus, thyroid disease, human immunodeficiency virus, pituitary disorders, long-term narcotic use, and obesity can all have an effect on testosterone levels, and including men with such comorbidities in studies can distort reported reference ranges.[3,42] Ultimately, whether reported reference ranges that have been established in healthy men are appropriate for men in various diseased states remains an area of active investigation.

Specifically, with regard to reference range variations related to differences in assay technologies, researchers have investigated ways to address these systemic differences and minimize their influence on reference range calculations. For example, normalizing equations derived through the harmonization of all measurements to a higher-order standard before the calculation of reference ranges have reduced intercohort variation of testosterone measurements, suggesting assay differences as major factors in observed geographical variations.[42] By cross-calibrating assays to a reference method and standard, these harmonized reference ranges can be applied across laboratories to reduce intercohort variations of testosterone measurements.[42]

Travison and colleagues[42] demonstrated the feasibility of harmonization procedures in a study that compared testosterone concentrations in 100 men from four cohorts in Europe and the United States: the Framingham Heart Study, the European Male Aging Study, the Osteoporotic Fractures in Men Study, and the Male Sibling Study of Osteoporosis. Travison and colleagues[42] were able to construct normalizing equations that generated harmonized values used to derive standardized, age-specific reference ranges by measuring testosterone concentrations calibrated to a higher-order benchmark, such as that provided by the CDC Reference Laboratory. A remarkable concordance in age-adjusted, harmonized testosterone levels among men in the four geographically distinct cohorts was demonstrated.[42] The harmonized normal reference range in a healthy, nonobese population of European and American men (aged 19–39 years) was reported to be 264 ng/dL–916 ng/dL (9.15–31.75 nmol/L).[42] Specifically, the harmonized 2.5th, 5th, 50th, 95th, and 97.5th percentile values were 264, 303, 531, 852, and 916 ng/dL, respectively.[42] This data from Travison and colleagues[42] demonstrate the feasibility and promise of calculating reference ranges using harmonized values that can be applied to laboratories that use calibrators such as those available from the National Institute of Standards and Technologies.

The application of reference ranges across laboratories and geographic regions has been and remains to be a formidable challenge. It not only requires mechanisms for the implementation of standardizing assays but also requires a fundamental understanding of the biological as well as social differences in analyte distribution. Furthermore, validation of the harmonized reference ranges using outcome-related data from randomized trials and longitudinal studies remains a complex yet crucial step in the clinical application of standardizing reference ranges.

OTHER FACTORS AFFECTING ACCURACY OF TOTAL TESTOSTERONE MEASUREMENT
Timing of Laboratory Testing

Circadian variation in testosterone levels is a well-documented phenomenon, with the highest levels of testosterone released in the morning and relatively lower levels of testosterone released in the afternoon and evening,[43] while trough levels of testosterone are observed approximately 12 hours after peak.[44] This diurnal variation in testosterone levels has been reported to be blunted in older populations of men. A 2009 study reported a 20–25% difference in testosterone levels in younger men (aged 30–40 years) between the hours of 08:00 and 16:00 compared to a 10% difference in testosterone levels between the same hours for older men (aged 70 years).[44]

Notably, this study of 66 men included many subjects with normal morning (before 12:00) testosterone levels ($\geq$300 ng/dL) and low testosterone levels (<300 ng/dL) in the afternoon. For these reasons, testosterone measurements should ideally be performed as close to waking as possible. In clinical practice, this may translate to sample procurement between 07:00 and 09:00.

Repeat Laboratory Testing

Testosterone laboratory values should be confirmed with at least one duplicate measurement for the diagnosis of low testosterone. In one community-based study, 30% of men with initial testosterone values considered to be in the hypogonadal range were found to have normal testosterone values on repeat measurements.[45] There has been evidence reported that week-to-week variability can account for some of this variation.[46] Another study, which employed frequent testing of testosterone levels at 20-minute intervals, found that 3 of 10 healthy subjects intermittently registered testosterone concentrations below the normal range.[47]

Repeat measurements have been noted to vary widely (65–153%) depending on the assay utilized. Conducting two or more repeat measurements can mitigate some of this variability.[45]

SUMMARY

Because the accurate diagnosis of male hypogonadism is dependent on the reliable assessment of testosterone levels, accurate detection and quantification of serum testosterone levels remains a necessary component of standard clinical care for the practicing urologist. Consensus guidelines routinely recommend that only men meeting criteria for TD should be offered TRT. The accurate quantification of testosterone levels remains a challenge, in part due to the diurnal fluctuations in serum testosterone, the wide range of normal testosterone values, and the technical as well as logistical challenges of performing assays. Although IAs and MS-based assays are commonly utilized in clinical practice, both these assay systems exhibit unique flaws that erroneously hinder the establishment of reference ranges. Moreover, reported reference ranges from distinct populations and cohorts cannot be applied more broadly to other populations around the world, but feasible measures, such as harmonization procedures, offer promise in the standardization of reference ranges.

CLINICS CARE POINT

- A diagnosis of hypogonadism should only be made in men with symptoms and signs consistent with testosterone deficiency and unequivocally low serum T concentrations on at least two early morning tests.
- The use of accurate assays for the measurement of testosterone and rigorously derived reference ranges for the interpretation of testosterone levels is necessary for the diagnosis of hypogonadism.

DISCLOSURE

The authors have nothing to disclose.

ACKNOWLEDGEMENT

The authors would like to thank Scott Bailey, PhD, for editing this manuscript.

REFERENCES

1. McEwan IJ, Brinkmann AO. Androgen Physiology: Receptor and Metabolic Disorders. 2021 Jul 2. In: Feingold KR, Anawalt B, Boyce A, et al, editors. Endotext [Internet]. South Dartmouth (MA): MDText.com, Inc.; 2000. PMID: 25905257.
2. Salter CA, Mulhall JP. Guideline of guidelines: testosterone therapy for testosterone deficiency. BJU Int 2019;124(5):722–9.
3. Mulhall JP, Trost LW, Brannigan RE, et al. Evaluation and management of testosterone deficiency: AUA guideline. J Urol 2018;200:423.
4. Vermeulen A, Verdonck L, Kaufman JM. A critical evaluation of simple methods for the estimation of free testosterone in serum. J Clin Endocrinol Metab 1999;84(10):3666–72.
5. Keevil BG, Adaway J. Assessment of free testosterone concentration. J Steroid Biochem Mol Biol 2019;190:207–11.
6. Rosner W. Sex steroids and the free hormone hypothesis. Cell 2006;124(3):455–6 [author reply: 456-7].
7. Goldman AL, Bhasin S, Wu FCW, et al. A Reappraisal of Testosterone's Binding in Circulation: Physiological and Clinical Implications. Endocr Rev 2017;38(4):302–24.
8. Pardridge WM. Serum bioavailability of sex steroid hormones. Clin Endocrinol Metab 1986;15(2):259–78.
9. Manni A, Pardridge WM, Cefalu W, et al. Bioavailability of albumin-bound testosterone. J Clin Endocrinol Metab 1985;61(4):705–10.
10. Nakhla AM, Leonard J, Hryb DJ, et al. Sex hormone-binding globulin receptor signal transduction proceeds via a G protein. Steroids 1999;64(3):213–6.
11. Lee DM, O'Neill TW, Pye SR, et al. The European Male Ageing Study (EMAS): design, methods, and recruitment. Int J Androl 2009;32(1):11–24.
12. Wu FC, Tajar A, Beynon JM, et al. Identification of Late-Onset Hypogonadism in Middle-Aged and Elderly Men. N Engl J Med, 363 2010;(2),:123–35.
13. Miller KK, Rosner W, Lee H, et al. Measurement of free testosterone in normal women and women with androgen deficiency: comparison of methods. J Clin Endocrinol Metab 2004;89(2):525–33.
14. Cao Z, Botelho J, Rej R, et al. Accuracy-based proficiency testing for testosterone measurements with immunoassays and liquid chromatography-mass spectrometry. Clin Chim Acta 2017;469:31–6.
15. Centers for Disease Control and Prevention. HoSt/VDSCP: Standardization of Measurement Procedures. CDC Hormone Standardization Program (CDC HoSt) Certified Total Testosterone Procedures. 2020. Available at: https://www.cdc.gov/labstandards/hs_standardization.html. Accessed February 5, 2022.
16. Herati AS, Cengiz C, Lamb DJ. Assays of Serum Testosterone. Urol Clin North Am 2016;43(2):177–84.
17. Wang C, Catlin DH, Demers LM, et al. Measurement of total serum testosterone in adult men: comparison of current laboratory methods versus liquid chromatography-tandem mass spectrometry. J Clin Endocrinol Metab 2004;89(2):534–43.
18. Taieb J, Mathian B, Millot F, et al. Testosterone measured by 10 immunoassays and by isotope-dilution gas chromatography-mass spectrometry in sera from 116 men, women, and children. Clin Chem 2003;49(8):1381–95.
19. Trost L, Mulhall J. Challenges in testosterone measurement, data interpretation, and methodological appraisal of interventional trials. J Sex Med 2017;13(7):1029–46.
20. Steinberger E, Ayala C, Hsi B. Utilization of commercial laboratory results in management of

hyperandrogenism in women. Endocr Pract 1998; 4:1–10.

21. Vesper HW, Bhasin S, Wang C, et al. Interlaboratory comparison study of serum total testosterone [corrected] measurements performed by mass spectrometry methods. Steroids 2009;74(6):498–503 [Epub 2009 Jan 30. Erratum in: Steroids. 2009 Sep;74(9):791. PMID: 19428438].

22. Kanakis GA, Tsametis CP, Goulis DG. Measuring testosterone in women and men. Maturitas 2019; 125:41–4.

23. Bhasin Shalender, Brito Juan P, Cunningham Glenn R, et al. Testosterone therapy in men with hypogonadism: an endocrine society clinical practice guideline. J Clin Endocrinol Metab 2018;103(5): 1715–44. https://doi.org/10.1210/jc.2018-00229. Available at:.

24. Kacker R, Hornstein A, Morgentaler A. Free testosterone by direct and calculated measurement versus equilibrium dialysis in a clinical population. Aging Male 2013;16(4):164–8.

25. Shea JL, Wong PY, Chen Y. Free testosterone: clinical utility and important analytical aspects of measurement. Adv Clin Chem 2014;63:59–84.

26. Vlahos I, MacMahon W, Sgoutas D, et al. An improved ultrafiltration method for determining free testosterone in serum. Clin Chem 1982;28(11): 2286–91. PMID: 7127776.

27. Chen Y, Yazdanpanah M, Wang XY, et al. Direct measurement of serum free testosterone by ultrafiltration followed by liquid chromatography tandem mass spectrometry. Clin Biochem 2010;43(4–5): 490–6.

28. Rosner W, Auchus RJ, Azziz R, et al. Position statement: Utility, limitations, and pitfalls in measuring testosterone: an Endocrine Society position statement. J Clin Endocrinol Metab 2007; 92(2):405–13.

29. Bhasin S, Cunningham GR, Hayes FJ, et al. Testosterone therapy in men with androgen deficiency syndromes: an Endocrine Society clinical practice guideline. J Clin Endocrinol Metab 2010;95(6): 2536–59 [Erratum in: J Clin Endocrinol Metab. 2021 Jun 16;106(7):e2848. PMID: 20525905].

30. Ho CKM, Stoddart M, Walton M, et al. Calculated free testosterone in men: comparison of four equations and with free androgen index. Ann Clin Biochem 2006;43:389–97.

31. Morris PD, Malkin CJ, Channer KS, et al. A mathematical comparison of techniques to predict biologically available testosterone in a cohort of 1072 men. Eur J Endocrinol 2004;151: 241–9.

32. Sartorius G, Ly LP, Sikaris K, et al. Predictive accuracy and sources of variability in calculated free testosterone estimates. Ann Clin Biochem 2009; 46(Pt 2):137–43.

33. Ly LP, Sartorius G, Hull L, et al. Accuracy of calculated free testosterone formulae in men. Clin Endocrinol (Oxf) 2010;73(3):382–8.

34. Yamamoto K, Koh E, Matsui F, et al. Measurement-specific bioavailable testosterone using concanavalin A precipitation: comparison of calculated and assayed bioavailable testosterone. Int J Urol 2009; 16(11):894–901.

35. Giton F, Guéchot J, Fiet J. Comparative determinations of non SHBG-bound serum testosterone, using ammonium sulfate precipitation, Concanavalin A binding or calculation in men. Steroids 2012; 77(12):1306–11.

36. Wang C, Nieschlag E, Swerdloff R, et al. Investigation, treatment and monitoring of late- onset hypogonadism in males: ISA, ISSAM, EAU, EAA and ASA recommendations. Eur J Endocrinol 2008;159: 507–14.

37. Bhasin S, Pencina M, Jasuja GK, et al. Reference ranges for testosterone in men generated using liquid chromatography tandem mass spectrometry in a community-based sample of healthy nonobese young men in the Framingham Heart Study and applied to three geographically distinct cohorts. J Clin Endocrinol Metab 2011; 96:2430–9.

38. Kaufman JM, Vermeulen A. The decline of androgen levels in elderly men and its clinical and therapeutic implications. Endocr Rev 2005;26(6):833–76.

39. Yeap BB, Alfonso H, Chubb SA, et al. Reference ranges and determinants of testosterone, dihydrotestosterone, and estradiol levels measured using liquid chromatography-tandem mass spectrometry in a population-based cohort of older men. J Clin Endocrinol Metab 2012;97(11):4030–9.

40. Livingston M, Kalansooriya A, Hartland AJ, et al. Serum testosterone levels in male hypogonadism: Why and when to check-A review. Int J Clin Pract 2017;71(11):e12995.

41. Feldman HA, Longcope C, Derby CA, et al. Age trends in the level of serum testosterone and other hormones in middle-aged men: longitudinal results from the Massachusetts male aging study. J Clin Endocrinol Metab 2002;87(2):589–98. https://doi.org/10.1210/jcem.87.2.8201.

42. Travison TG, Vesper HW, Orwoll E, et al. Harmonized reference ranges for circulating testosterone levels in men of four cohort studies in the united states and Europe. J Clin Endocrinol Metab 2017;102(4): 1161–73.

43. Pastuszak AW, Gittelman M, Tursi JP, et al. Pharmacokinetics of testosterone therapies in relation to diurnal variation of serum testosterone levels as men age. Andrology 2021. https://doi.org/10.1111/andr.13108.

44. Brambilla DJ, Matsumoto AM, Araujo AB, et al. The effect of diurnal variation on clinical measurement

of serum testosterone and other sex hormone levels in men. J Clin Endocrinol Metab 2009;94(3):907–13.

45. Brambilla DJ, O'Donnell AB, Matsumoto AM, et al. Intraindividual variation in levels of serum testosterone and other reproductive and adrenal hormones in men. Clin Endocrinol (Oxf) 2007;67(6): 853–62.

46. Morley JE, Patrick P, Perry HM 3rd. Evaluation of assays available to measure free testosterone. Metabolism 2002;51(5):554–9.

47. Spratt DI, O'Dea LS, Schoenfeld D, et al. Neuroendocrine-gonadal axis in men: frequent sampling of LH, FSH, and testosterone. Am J Phys 1988;254(5 Pt 1):E658–66.

Testosterone Replacement Options

Andrew Richard McCullough, MD[a,*], Mehvish Khan, MD[b]

KEYWORDS

- Testosterone • Testosterone injections • Testosterone gels and patches • Testosterone therapies
- Nasal testosterone • Buccal testosterone • Oral testosterone

KEY POINTS

- There is a plethora of different testosterone replacement options, each with their own advantages and disadvantages.
- Long-term adherence to testosterone therapy is poor, reflecting unrealistic patient expectations and understanding of the benefits, poor follow-up, provider difficulty with the choice of modality, understanding pharmacologic differences between the modalities.
- Understanding the physiology of hypogonadism and the pharmacokinetics of each preparation is important for the practitioner to understand to make the right choice for each patient.

INTRODUCTION

Testosterone plays a critical role in the regulation of male sexual, somatic and behavioral functions important to lifelong well-being. Testosterone deficiency is a consequence of reduced testosterone production because of hypothalamic-pituitary-gonadal axis pathology or senescence. Hypogonadism, which can be multifactorial, is diagnosed based on a constellation of clinical symptoms and signs and confirmed biochemically by documentation of consistently low serum total testosterone levels.

The treatment of hypogonadism by medical providers can be challenging. Owing to market development and availability of no less than 15 treatment options, both clinicians and patients must decide on the optimal formulation by taking multiple factors into consideration including cost, mode of delivery, ease of use, compliance, and the pharmacokinetics of each preparation. The provider and patient must navigate conflicting scientific evidence about the definition of hypogonadism and indications for treatment, uncertain target clinical and biochemical endpoints, the ambiguity of benefits and risks, regulatory constraints, the overabundance of media hype and internet marketing with its attendant misinformation, the lack of formal education during training in male hypogonadism and the confusing number of options of treatment and schedules of administration. The purpose of this article was to review the physiology of hypogonadism and the differences between the current treatment modalities to equip the reader with the tools to make thoughtful choices among the multitude of modalities available in the treatment of hypogonadism.

PHYSIOLOGY

In order to understand the therapy of hypogonadism, it is important to understand the basic physiology of endogenous testosterone production.

Testosterone Production and Transport

Testosterone is an anabolic steroid that is derived from cholesterol. More than 95% is synthesized in the mitochondria and endoplasmic reticulum of the Leydig cells of the testes, under the regulation of pituitary gonadotropin LH, and the remainder is produced in the adrenal glands. The daily production is between 3 to 11 mg per day.[1] Testosterone

[a] Department of Urology, Beth Israel Lahey Medical Center, 41 Mall Road, Burlington, MA 01805, USA;
[b] Division of Endocrinology, Beth Israel Lahey Medical Center, 41 Mall Road, Burlington, MA 01805, USA
* Corresponding author.
E-mail address: Andrew.mccullough@lahey.org

Urol Clin N Am 49 (2022) 679–693
https://doi.org/10.1016/j.ucl.2022.07.010
0094-0143/22/© 2022 Elsevier Inc. All rights reserved.

urologic.theclinics.com

has a short half-life of 10 to 100 min. LH stimulates testosterone production in a pulsatile fashion, with peaks every one to 3 h. With age, both the frequency and the amplitude of the pulses decrease. In addition, the Leydig cells become less responsive to LH, and their total number decreases with age.[2] Given the short half-life of testosterone, the frequency of natural LH pulses is not surprising.

Testosterone is transported in the serum, tightly bound to sex-hormone-binding globulin (SHBG) (~70%) and loosely bound to albumin (~30%). Approximately 2% is totally free. The SHBG molecule is produced by the liver and binds two testosterone molecules. Typically, SHBG is close to equimolar to testosterone (20 nmoles/L). An abnormally high SHBG, can result in a low free testosterone despite what might seem like a normal total testosterone. In a patient with cirrhosis or hepatitis, the SHBG levels can exceed 100 nmoles/L. For such a patient to have a mid-range calculated free testosterone level, his total testosterone would have to be more than 1000 ng/dL. As men age, their SHBG increases, sometimes resulting in low free testosterone levels with total testosterone levels in the normal range. Other conditions associated with increased SHBG are hyperthyroidism, use of anticonvulsants, use of estrogens or HIV disease.[3]

Testosterone Metabolism

Testosterone is metabolized hepatically and peripherally. It is metabolized into active and inactive metabolites. The two active metabolites produced are dihydrotestosterone (5%–8%) and estradiol (0.3%–5%) by the 5α-reductase and aromatase enzymatic systems, respectively.[4] The 5α-reductase enzymes are found in the prostate and skin and the aromatase enzymes are found in the peripheral fat tissue and testis.

The hepatic cytochrome P450 system is responsible approximately 95% of the metabolism of testosterone through a series of inactivating hydroxylation reactions followed by glucuronidation and to a lesser extent sulfation. The hydrophilic conjugates are excreted in the urine and bile.[5] Less than 5% of testosterone is excreted unchanged in the urine. Medications, medical conditions or inherent individual biodiversity of the cytochrome P450 system can significantly increase or decrease the half-life of testosterone.

The first pass absorption of oral testosterone from the liver and intestine is rapid, as is the clearance. Testosterone injected intravenously has been shown to have a half-life of less than 60 min.[6] The efficient absorption of oral testosterone and its rapid clearance make replacement

with oral non-esterified testosterone impractical. To counter the rapid metabolism, esterification of the molecule is necessary.

Testosterone Natural Biologic Activity

The endogenous natural biological activity of testosterone is complex and can be affected by the concentration of testosterone, the differential expression of the androgen receptor in the target tissue types, polymorphism of the androgen receptor, the concentration of androgen binding hormones produced in the liver and testes, tissue-specific levels of 5α-reductase and aromatase enzymes, and tissue-specific levels of androgen receptor (AR) promoters.[7] This may partly explain why different symptoms of hypogonadism (sexual dysfunction vs muscle strength) respond to different levels of testosterone replacement.[8]

Classical and Non-classical Mechanism of Action

Testosterone has both genomic (classical) and non-genomic actions (non-classical). Classical action mediates its effects via a cytoplasmic ligand-dependent nuclear transcription factor AR. The AR is expressed to different degrees in a diverse range of tissues including bone, muscle, prostate, adipose tissue, and the reproductive, cardiovascular, neural, and hematopoietic systems. Testosterone exerts its genomic effect by binding to the AR to regulate target gene transcription. The genomic signaling, also referred to as the DNA binding-dependent action of the AR, occurs when androgens bind to the AR leading to a conformational change in the receptor and translocation of the androgen-AR complex into the nucleus. This complex with promoters then binds to the specific androgen response elements (AREs) within target genes via the DNA binding domain (DBD) of the AR to modulate gene transcription and translation.

Non-genomic effects are rapidly occurring when the androgen-AR complex at the cell membrane level. This complex activates kinase signaling cascades and initiates initiating phosphorylation of a second messenger signaling cascade. In addition, activation of membrane-bound protein receptors such as G-protein coupled receptor and iron-regulated transported like protein 9 (ZIP9) can trigger intracellular signaling pathways.[7,9–11] It is important for the reader to understand that the differential contribution of genomic vs non-genomic effects on clinical presentation is not understood.

General principles
Conditions for treatment Over the last many years, there has been an increase in testosterone

prescriptions with many men using testosterone without a clear indication, criteria, or appropriate follow-up. As per American Urological Association (AUA), the clinical diagnosis of testosterone deficiency is made when patients have both consistently low morning testosterone levels less than 300 ng/dL combined with signs and symptoms of androgen deficiency symptoms including decreased libido, erectile dysfunction, hot flashes, loss of muscle mass, weakness, weight gain, depressed mood, and loss of muscle mass or hair loss. The endocrine society (ES) recommends evaluating hypogonadal men with incomplete or delayed sexual development, eunuchoidism, reduced sexual desire (libido) and activity, decreased spontaneous erections, breast discomfort, gynecomastia, loss of body (axillary and pubic) hair, reduced shaving, very small testes, inability to father children, low or zero sperm count, height loss, low trauma fracture, low bone mineral density, and hot flushes or sweats.[3] Both societies recommend two morning fasting testosterone measurements. **Table 1**.

Are morning testosterones necessary? When to measure testosterone levels? Serum testosterone levels can show a day-to-day and long-term biologic variation, as well as a diurnal variation. In a random sample of 132 asymptomatic men in the Boston Area Community, the majority of whom were eugonadal, the day-to-day and long-term biologic variation ranged from 18% to 54%.[12] The same group of authors reported age-related diurnal variations in 66 asymptomatic healthy men (ages 30–80). In men between 30 and 40, testosterone declined 20% to 25% whereas in men aged 70 the decline was only 10%.[13] Of note is that most studies for testosterone variability are done on healthy volunteers. In a study of the circadian variation in 859 hypogonadal men (T_{mean} 239 ng/dL), a blunted diurnal variation was seen, the mean amplitude was 32.4 ng/dL. Even at the T peak level, the hypogonadal men remained hypogonadal.[14] In a retrospective "single draw" study of 2569 men with erectile dysfunction Kohler showed no difference in mean TT at any time between 7 AM and 2 PM in men older than 45.[15]

The regulatory approval of a TRT product is based on achieving a level of testosterone between 300 and 100 ng/dL in at least 75% of men with a diagnosis of hypogonadism ($T < 300$ ng/dL) irrespective of any symptom improvement.[16] All the TRT registry trials were conducted based on two a.m. blood draws showing hypogonadism in order to maximize uniformity. Both AUA and ESA guidelines, therefore, recommend two a.m.

blood draws to establish the diagnosis of hypogonadism. Following the guidelines, third-party payers mandate two morning blood draws before approval of insurance coverage. It is important to realize that the choice of a.m. blood draws in clinical trials was arbitrary and one of convenience for the clinical trial staff.

Fasting measurements or not? Testosterone measurements in all the registry trials were done in a fasting state to ensure uniformity. Food intake may suppress serum testosterone concentrations. In a cross-sectional study of 74 eugonadal men aged 37 to 51, glucose ingestion induced a significant reduction in total and free T levels due a direct testicular defect. There was an absence of compensatory response in LH which suggested an alternative central component.[17] Another study done in Sweden compared testosterone levels after overnight fasting to levels measured 60 to 120 min after a standard meal and a decline of testosterone level of 30% was noted.[18] This study also did not find a change in LH or SHBG levels. The effect of food has not been extensively studied in symptomatic hypogonadal men. Fasting should be considered by the practitioner to maximize uniformity of measurements. An early morning draw does not guarantee a fasting state.

Goals for treatment The goal of testosterone therapy is the normalization of total testosterone levels along with improvement in some of the symptoms. Unfortunately, many of these symptoms are vague, difficult to quantitative, multifactorial, and sometimes just associated with aging and the stress of life. The AUA guidelines conditionally recommend using the minimal dosing necessary to bring testosterone levels in the mid tertile of the normal reference range (450–600), whereas the ES suggests a target value to be the mid-range for a normal young man. The exact serum testosterone levels required to achieve optimal efficacy and safety are currently unknown.

When to evaluate therapeutic levels The AUA recommends follow-up lab testing between 2 to 4 weeks after initiation of therapy and then every 6 to 12 months to assess serum testosterone levels, symptomatic improvement, prostate-specific antigen (PSA), and changes in hematocrit (Hct). The ES recommends follow-up 3 months after initiation of TTh and then every 6 to 12 months thereafter. The distinct PK profile of each testosterone formulation accounts for the specific timing when testosterone levels should be measured in reference to the dosage to allow for dose adjustments and monitoring. This is mainly influenced by the way the clinical trials are designed and

Table 1
AUA and Endocrine Society guidelines

Guidelines	AUA[19]	ES[3]
When to measure T	AM fasting total T x 2	AM fasting total T x 2
Normal range total T	450–600 ng/dL	264–916 ng/dL
Biochemical T deficiency	<300 ng/dL	<264 ng/dL
Aim	Middle tertile of normal range and improvement in symptoms/signs	Mid-normal range for young men and improvement in symptoms/signs
First therapeutic evaluation	2–4 wk	3 mo
Long-term follow-up	6–12 mo	6–12 mo

conducted. For most of the gel forms, including Androgel 1% and 1.62%, Testim 1%, and Vogelxo, the levels are measured before the morning dose. Fortesta is an exception, in which the levels are measured 2 h after application based on its specific PK profile. The logic for the recommended testing schedule is not clear (**Table 2**). If an Hct level increases to greater than 54%, treatment options include discontinuation of TTh, therapeutic phlebotomy, or consideration of switching to another testosterone formulation.[19]

Therapeutic success challenges Although testosterone replacement has the potential to improve symptoms, continuation of therapy is a major problem. Factors contributing to discontinuations are cost, lack of perceived benefit, inconvenience of the administration, inconvenience to the provider. In a British Columbia study, 40% of men discontinued treatment after their first or second treatment and only 27% had 10 or more repeated prescriptions. From a prescriber's perspective, only 36% of patients had post-treatment testosterone levels documented. Primary care and Urologists were responsible for 86% and 5% of prescriptions with gels and injectables accounting for roughly 50% each.[20] In studies of gel therapy adherence to treatment ranged from 15% to 19% at 1 year with no difference between the brands.[20–22] The adherence to short-lasting IM T injections is no better despite arguably higher testosterone levels.[23] Although adherence to office-based therapies such as subcutaneous (SC) pellets, monthly injections, and long-acting TU is high for men who present to the office therapy dropout rates are significant because of the inconvenience of the office visits and associated visit co-payments.

Unrealistic patient expectations The reason men seek testosterone therapy vary and can include well-being, low energy, libido, and erectile dysfunction.[24] Many men are self-diagnosed, getting their information through advertising and the internet where as few as 30% of the websites are deemed to be "high quality," at an appropriate grade level and contain comprehensive information as to the risks and benefits.[25] In older men with organic vasculogenic erectile dysfunction, lack of improvement in erectile function may be perceived by the patient as a treatment failure. Similarly, lack of improvement in energy level, sense of well-being, and obesity despite not addressing lifestyle changes as well can be perceived as treatment failure. It is important for the clinician to have a clear understanding of the symptom being treated and to portray realistic outcomes.

Costs Costs are frequently quoted as a reason for discontinuation Most testosterone therapies can be provided in generic form at great savings to the patients. With proper documentation by the provider (ie, Two a.m. testosterone levels less than 300 ng/dL) most insurance companies will cover treatment. Whereas more expensive non-generic treatments may not be included in a plan or have exorbitant co-payments, generic treatments are generally covered. Many providers are not aware of the inexpensive nature of generic testosterone, frequently falling below co-pay levels for the medication levied by the insurer. Through internet websites, the consumer can frequently find prices that are heavily discounted. The web-based companies partner with the pharmacies to provide competitive pricing and deep discounts helping to make a dent in the problem of medication non-adherence.[26] The price per month if out of pocket can vary from low as $11 to $955 depending on the preparation. **Table 3** is a list of the self-pay costs through the web-based company GoodRx. Eleven dollars a month is affordable to most patients.

Provider barriers

A schedule III drug: Testosterone is a schedule III drug subject to the same reporting laws as

Table 2
When to measure serum testosterone levels for monitoring

Testosterone Formulations	Timing of Testosterone Measurement
Gels[a]	Morning preapplication level
Androgel® 1% and 1.62%	Morning preapplication level
Testim® 1%	2 h after application
Fortesta® 2%	Predose
Volgelxo®	
Patches	12 h after application
Androderm®	
Intranasal	2 h after application
Natesto®	
Oral	6 h after morning dose
JATENZO®	
Pellets	End of dosing interval
Testopel®	
Intramuscular injections	Mid-way between the two injections
Testosterone Enanthate and	
Testosterone Cypionate	
Subcutaneous Injections	Trough concentrations (measured 7 d after most recent dose) obtained following 6 wk of dosing
Xyosted®	
Long-acting subcutaneous injection	Mid-way between the two 10-wk injections
AVEED®®	

[a] Levels are measured at nadir, with the exception of Fortesta.

opiates. All prescriptions get reported to a prescription monitoring program (PMP) in all states. Most states mandate electronic prescribing and limit the number of refills to 6 months. Some states require monthly electronic prescriptions forcing the provider to write 12 prescriptions a year for every patient on testosterone therapy. Depending on the electronic medical record system, 7 mouse clicks may be required with an entry of a multicharacter user identification code for every prescription, not to mention the need to check safety labs before each prescription and adherence to semiannual or annual visits, as per guidelines. These prescriptions cannot be delegated to nonmedically licensed personnel, and the administrative time is non-reimbursable. On the other hand, adherence to therapy is easily monitored through PMP websites.

Prior authorization: Every new prescription submitted to insurance companies is subject to a prior authorization which requires two morning testosterone blood draws to document hypogonadism. This administrative burden can be delegated to a medical assistant but is still time-consuming and incurs a practice cost.

Nonbillable visit and financial liabilities: The SC pellets and long-acting TU IM shots each require 30 min of office time and 3 to 5 visits a year just to deliver a scheduled treatment. As such, Evaluation and Management codes are frequently denied. The federally mandated 6% withhold for Medicare patients results in a financial loss for the pellets or TU if they are purchased by the practice. Nonpayment by insurance or the patient for one treatment of either can easily result in a $1000 loss, by far offsetting the insertion or insertion or injection fee.

Compliance Clinicians should discuss the cessation of testosterone therapy three to 6 months after commencement of treatment in patients who experience normalization of total testosterone levels but fail to achieve symptom or sign improvement.[19] Before discontinuation, though, it is incumbent on the practitioner to ascertain whether the patient is compliant with the therapy. The patient's behavior in sponsor-supported clinical trials is not always reflected in real-life experience. In a clinical trial, compliance is monitored, regular blood draws are rigorously scheduled, the

Table 3 Self pay costs on GoodRx website	
Testosterone prep	**30 d ($)**
Testosterone enanthate 5 mLs (1000 mgs) multiuse vial	11–22
Testosterone cypionate 4 mL (800 mgs) single use vials	27–86
Androgel® Pump 1.62% generic	38–145
Androgel® Pump 1% generic	54–86
Androgel® Packets 50 mgs generic	90–188
Vogelxo® pump 1%	104–361
Vogelxo® packets generic	120–361
Natesto®® (5.5 mg/actuation)	193–305
Xyosted® (50 mg)	456–572
Xyosted® (75 mg)	456–572
Xyosted® (100 mg)	456–572
Testim® packets Brand	590–616
Androgel® pump 1.62% Brand	619–646
Androgel® packets 50 mg Brand	638–666
JATENZO® (237 mg BID)	955

medication is provided by the sponsor and there is frequently a non-coercive financial incentive for continuation. Unrealistic expectations, faulty and sporadic supplication of gels, patches, missed injection or insertion appointments, missed self-injections, delay in prescription refills and renewals and financial pressures can all result in therapeutic failure unrelated to the efficacy of the modality chosen. Patients may not be regularly compliant yet apply their gel the morning of a blood draw, giving the practitioner a false sense of compliance. As testosterone is a schedule III drug, compliance and timing of refills can be checked through the PMP, just as for narcotics. Adding to the confusion as to biochemical efficacy is the variability of when the blood measurements are taken. Although the guidelines specify when testing should be done after treatment is started, the timing of the blood draws varies for each modality. Each formulation has a different PK profile. The timing of labs should be tailored to each individual mode of therapy. Some measurements are recommended at the peak, some mid-cycle, and some at the nadir[27] (see **Table 2**). The pharmacokinetic properties of each modality should be taken into consideration.

TESTOSTERONE PREPARATIONS
Topical/Transdermal

Gels
General principles
- All dermal gels are poorly absorbed. Only 10% to 15% of the gel applied is bioavailable.

The rest remains on the body until it is washed off
- Secondary exposure: To prevent inadvertent exposure of women and children to testosterone gels, patients are instructed to wash their hands after using the product. Treated sites are covered with clothing once the gel has dried and to wash treated skin areas if skin-skin contact is anticipated. Currently, all testosterone liquids and gels in the United States contain a US Food and Drug Administration (FDA) warning for the risk of transference.
- Daily application is mandatory as levels return to baseline at 48 h.
- Gonadotropin levels were suppressed in the registry trials. Failure to find suppressed levels despite good T levels in follow-up suggests poor compliance. Failure to find suppressed levels with poor T levels suggests poor application technique, poor absorption, or noncompliance with the application.

Three testosterone gels are available: Androgel, Testim, and Fortesta.

Androgel: Androgel was the first gel and became available in June 2000. Androgel is a hydroalcoholic formulation. It is available in 1% and 1.62% concentrations. The 1% concentration is available in packets and metered-dose pump bottles. The packets contain either 25 mg/2.5 g or 50 mg/5 g of testosterone, whereas the pump delivers 12.5 mg of testosterone per actuation. The starting dose of Androgel 1% is 50 mg. Areas of application include shoulders, upper arms, or abdomen. A patient can swim or shower after 5 h with Androgel 1%. A randomized, parallel study of 227 hypogonadal men evaluated the pharmacokinetics of the Androgel 1% and compared gel 50 mg/d to gel 100 mg/d [28] The C_{max} occurred 18 to 24 h after application and the C_{min} occurred 8 to 12 h later. A steady state is achieved by the second or third day of dosing. The levels return to baseline 48 to 72 h after applying the gel. The levels were measured prior to the morning application.

The Androgel 1.62% preparation is also available packets and metered-dose pump bottles. The unit dose packets contain either 20.25 mg/1.25 g or 50.5 mg/2.5 g of testosterone. The metered-dose pump provides 20.25 mg of testosterone per actuation of 1.25 g of gel. The starting dose of Androgel is 1.62% is 40.5 mg daily. A patient can swim or shower and after 2 h with Androgel 1.62%. Areas of application include shoulders and upper arms. It is not indicated to be applied to the abdomen. A study with 36 male subjects compared the bioavailability of this preparation at different sites. The study showed 30%–40% lower availability when it was applied to the abdomen than to the arms and shoulders.[29]

Adverse effects specific to Androgel include acne, application site reaction, and increased PSA level.[27]

Testim was approved by FDA in February 2003. Testim is a 1% gel supplied in 5 and 10 g tubes which contain 50 and 100 mg of testosterone, respectively. The starting dose is 50 mg in the morning, but some patients can be titrated to two tubes, or 100 mg of testosterone. Testim is to be applied on the shoulders and upper arms. Testim has been shown to have enhanced absorption and serum testosterone levels due to the presence of the penetration enhancer, pentadectalactone, which is found in many aftershaves and colognes leading to a musk-like odor with its application.[30] Median T_{max} of Testim is 18 h and average serum concentration levels are achieved within 24 h.[31] Levels are measured in the morning after initiation. Patients can swim or shower 2 h after applying Testim. Up to 4% of the patients can experience injection site reaction when using the 100 mg dose of Testim.

Fortesta was approved by the FDA in 2010. Fortesta is a 2% gel that contains oleic acid, a known penetration enhancer. It is supplied in a metered dose pump. Each pump delivers only 0.5 g of gel containing 10 mg testosterone. The starting dose is 4 pump actuations (40 mg) applied topically to the front or inner thighs daily in the morning. The dose can be titrated to 70 mg. The effects of Fortesta 2% gel on serum testosterone levels was evaluated in a multicenter, open-label study of 129 men with hypogonadism.[32] The subjects applied Fortesta 2%, 40 mg/d for 90 days and 77.5% of patients had C_{avg} at 90 days, similar to levels on day 35. Testosterone peaked at 2 to 4 h after application and fell to baseline levels 12 h after application. Also, another study conducted on 34 patients showed normal testosterone levels within 3 h with a steady state being achieved at a median time of 1.1 days. Furthermore, it showed that the gel dries in less than 3 min after application.[33] The levels in these studies were measured 2 h post application. Patients can swim or shower after 2 h. Treatment-related side effects included skin dryness.[27] The clinical trials excluded BMI > 35 and age >75.

Vogelxo TEVA was approved in 1953 and is made in Canada. It is available in unit dose packets, tube, or metered dose pumps. The starting dose is 50 mg of testosterone (one tube or one packet or 4 pump actuations) applied at the same time daily to the shoulders or upper arms.

Testosterone concentrations are measured pre-dose to adjust the dosing. The most common side effects are application site reaction, increased blood pressure, and headache.

Axiron: This is a 2% solution. The FDA posted a notice regarding the discontinuation of the manufacture of Axiron in September 2017. The product was not discontinued or withdrawn for safety or efficacy reasons but because of the multiple manufacturers that currently supply the US market.

Patches Androderm
General principles
- Following patch application, T_{max} is at approximately 8 h
- Nadir is achieved within 24 h of patch removal
- The patch is applied at night to mimic normal circadian pattern and the testosterone levels are measured in the morning, 12 h after the application which may not reflect nadir levels
- Skin rash is the most observed adverse effect leading to discontinuation of its use

Transdermal delivery of testosterone first became available in 1994 in the form of a scrotal patch. These were later discontinued because of scrotal irritation and application challenges and are no longer available in the United States.[27]

Androderm: This was FDA approved in 1995. This patch is available in 2 or 4 mg/d formulations. Based on pharmacokinetic analysis of the 5 g patch (which is no longer available), the T_{max} concentration averaged 765 ng/dL and occurred 8.2 h after \ application. The mean T_{min} was 280 ng/dL. The time-average concentration (C_{avg}) over the 24-h dosing interval was 517 ng/dL.[34] Following application, testosterone is continuously absorbed during the 24-h dosing period with a median (range) T_{max} of 8 (4–12) h and hypogonadal concentrations are achieved within 24 h of patch removal.[35] This has an apparent half-life of 1.3 h.[27] A higher rate of testosterone delivery is observed during the first 12 h ($\sim$60% of the total) compared with that during the second 12 h. The starting dose is 4 mg patch every 24 h at night at 10 PM to produce physiologic concentrations and mimic normal circadian pattern, the importance of which is questionable in an older man. By applying the patch at night testosterone levels will be lowest at the end of the day, when many men describe their hypogonadal symptoms. The patches can be applied to the back, abdomen, thighs, or upper arms, The patches should be applied daily and sites should be rotated and not re-used within 7 days.[35] Testosterone levels are measured in the morning, 12 h after application of the patch the night prior.[34]

Approximately 30% of men who try this preparation are not able to continue with it because of severe skin rash. Some studies have found that pretreating with 1% triamcinolone acetonide cream applied under the patch can decrease the risk of dermatitis without compromising testosterone absorption. Some men have found benefits in applying hydrocortisone cream on the affected area after removal of the patch. Other adverse reactions include pruritis, skin induration, vesicle formation, allergic contact dermatitis, headaches, and depression. The patient should avoid showering, swimming, or washing the site for at least 3 h after application.[35]

Intranasal gels Natesto
General principles
- Absorption is rapid, with T_{max} occurring at 1 h, requiring multiple daily doses to achieve adequate levels of testosterone
- Levels fluctuate widely in a 24-h period with long periods at hypogonadal levels
- Meant to "mimic" normal circadian variation of testosterone levels throughout the day which is depicted by decreased LH and FSH levels 2 h after dosing with eventual recovery
- TID compliance is problematic and long-term adherence to therapy is questionable
- Replacement strategy with the least effect on sperm count and hematocrit

Natesto was approved by the FDA in 2014 and is the first intranasal testosterone to become available in the United States. It is available as a metered dose pump and each pump actuation gel contains 5.5 mg of testosterone in 122.5 mg of gel. The recommended dose is 11 mg 3 times daily. The nasal mucosa offers high permeability and high bioavailability, as the drug is not subject to first-pass metabolism[36,37].

Over 2 decades ago, an open, randomized, multiple-dose, study of 8 hypogonadal men in Romania tested an intranasal gel containing 7.6, 15.2, and 22.8 g of testosterone which showed that the maximum serum concentration of testosterone was achieved within 1 to 2 h indicating a rapid absorption from the intranasal cavity. It was also noted that the exposure to exogenous testosterone increased approximately linearly between 7.6 and 15.2 mg but leveled off with the higher dose of 22.8 mg likely because of the restricted volume for nasal application reflecting a saturation phenomenon at the site of absorption. Because of the rapid absorption with single dose nasal gel, multiple daily doses are required to achieve appropriate levels of testosterone which is meant to more closely proximate the normal circadian variation of testosterone levels throughout the day in a young man.

Natesto was evaluated in a more recent multicenter, open-label, 90-day clinical study that enrolled 306 men and randomly assigned them to either twice or thrice daily treatments. Intranasal Testosterone gel was self-administered using a multiple dose dispenser consistent with 5.5 mg testosterone per nostril, for a total of 11.0 mg single dose. PK studies were done based on predose samples collected on days 30 and 90. The T_{max} of testosterone appears at about 1 h, followed by a return to endogenous, predose levels 4 to 6 h later.[38] The $C_{average}$ testosterone was 421 ng/dL. The $C_{average}$ reflected the high peak levels, as testosterone levels dropped to baseline within 4 h. LH and FSH levels measured in this study at 2 h after dosing in all instances were decreased compared with baseline however they remained in the normal range. It seems that following this temporal suppression, the levels recovered over time. A study analyzing the preservation of spermatogenesis showed that mean sperm counts were unchanged after 6 months of nasal testosterone treatment in TID dosing. The lack of gonadotropin and sperm count suppression begs the question of the necessity of the maintenance of high levels of testosterone in the treatment of hypogonadism. A placebo randomized controlled trial of nasal testosterone on symptomatic hypogonadal men would be necessary to answer that question. Erythrocytosis was rare as 8 of 306 subjects (2.6%) had Hct values $\geq$ 54%.[39] Adverse reactions include increased PSA, headache, rhinorrhea, epistaxis, nasal discomfort, nasopharyngitis, upper respiratory tract infection (URI), sinusitis, bronchitis, and nasal scab formation[40]

The long-term compliance of TID dosing for short-term medications has been shown to be far inferior to once-a-day dosing.[41] With long-term compliance with once-daily gels being as low as 15%, it is hard to imagine good long-term compliance with TID dosing of Natesto. Long-term prescription data will answer that question.

Oral testosterone JATENZO
General principles
- Low bioavailability due to first-pass hepatic and intestinal metabolism
- Low bioavailability is illustrated in the requirement of large doses of twice daily TU to achieve therapeutic efficacy
- Higher bioavailability is achieved when taken with a fat-containing meal
- Dose adjustments are based on serum levels measured 6 h after the morning dose and do not reflect the nadir levels

- Most expensive therapy with poor insurance coverage
- BID dosing may present a compliance problem

When administered orally, testosterone is subject to significant inactivation in the GI tract and the liver. Adding an alkyl group in the 17-alpha position of testosterone slows its metabolism. In 1975 investigators reported that whereas orally administered free testosterone was not found to increase serum testosterone, esterified testosterone with the 9 carbon undecanoate chain resulted in increases in serum testosterone.[42] It was subsequently shown in four patients in whom their thoracic ducts were cannulated, that orally administered radioactively labeled TU appeared simultaneously in the lymph and serum two to 5 h after the dose was given and subsequently, 2 h after the peak serum levels it appeared in the urine. At 24 h 40% of the administered dose was excreted in the urine, predominantly as testosterone and androsterone-glucuronide. The authors postulated that TU was partially absorbed in the small intestine and absorbed in the lymphatic system and that 100% of the systemically available testosterone ester was lymphatically transported.[43] In March 2019, FDA approved JATENZO, a gelatin oral capsule (158 mg/198 mg/237 mg) containing testosterone undecanoate to be used for patients with hypogonadism. It is lipophilic and is absorbed via the intestinal lymphatic system but is subject to the first pass intestinal and hepatic metabolism. The oral bioavailability is estimated at 7%.[44] The low bioavailability is reflected in the large doses of twice-daily TU to achieve therapeutic efficacy (**Tables 4** and **5**). To promote lymphatic absorption the medication is best taken immediately before breakfast and dinner. The fat content of the meals was found to impact testosterone levels. When JATENZO was dosed with different breakfasts containing various amounts of fat, the bioavailability with the 30 g fat, 45 g fat, and high-calorie high-fat breakfasts was comparable, but there a negative food impact was seen with the 15 g (135 cal) fat breakfast (roughly equivalent to 2 tablespoons of peanut butter) compared with the 30 g (270 cal) fat breakfast. The 15 g fat breakfast had a 25% decrease in testosterone exposure compared with the 30 g fat breakfast. Intake conditions can have a 10-fold impact on T levels and can play a major role in intra- and inter-individual variability of testosterone levels.[45,46]

Efficacy was shown in a 4-month open-label comparator trial involving 166 men on JANENZO and 44 men on the topical gel. Eighty-seven percent of men achieved a daily C_{avg} in the normal range. C_{avg} level achieved was 403 ng/dL. Mean LH and FSH levels decreased 70% from baseline, comparable to the comparator topical T gel group. T_{min} dropped to baseline hypogonadal levels between 9 to 12 and 22 to 24 after dosing. Dose adjustments are therefore recommended based on serum testosterone 6 h after the morning dose and 7 days after starting the therapy. Clinicians outside of a clinical trial setting must make sure that blood draws are mid-to-late afternoon after a healthy breakfast.[44] Seminal parameters were not examined. The 24-h average increase in systolic BP was 4.9 mm Hg and an average HCT increase of 6%. No liver toxicity was detected.

Despite the lack of transference and the convenience of the oral dosing vs injections, the low bioavailability, dependence of testosterone levels on fat ingestion, twice-daily dosing, and expense make this a challenging modality for compliance and adherence to therapy.

Parenteral Testosterone Preparations

Intramuscular injections
General principles
- Oldest testosterone product
- FDA package insert is anachronistic, confusing, and does not reflect the pharmacokinetics of the product
- Least expensive with self-administration
- Most painful administration leading to poor long-term adherence to therapy
- Modality with maximum dosage variability
- Highest rate of erythrocytosis

Currently available long-acting injections include testosterone enanthate and testosterone cypionate. These synthetic compounds of testosterone have been made more lipophilic by the esterification of a fatty acid to the 17-beta hydroxyl group, thereby allowing for a longer duration of action. Owing to the high viscosity of the oils intramuscular (IM) injections are recommended in package insert. Dosing schedule is confusing at 50 mg to 400 mg every one to 4 weeks. Owing to the exponential decay after injection, a 4-week injection results in wide fluctuation of levels with early supratherapeutic levels followed by subtherapeutic testosterone levels toward the end of the treatment period. As testosterone is distributed evenly throughout the whole body an obese man is likely to require more testosterone. With exponential decay during the treatment period, mid-cycle testosterone measurements may overestimate the levels at the end of the treatment period. In general, lower doses more frequently result in

Table 4
Daily dosing

Testosterone Formulation	Dose (mg)	mg/d
Nasal	11	33
Subcutaneous Pellets	150–450	0.83–3.75
Transdermal patch	4	4
Gels	40–50	40–50
IM T Cypionate	50–400/2–4 wk	3.6–14
IM T Enanthate	100–400/1–4 wk	3.6–14
IM T Undecanoate	750/10 wk	27–18.75
SC T Enanthate	50/75/100	7–14
Oral T Undecanoate	158/198/237	316–474

more stable levels but the frequent IM injections are poorly tolerated by patients.

Testosterone cypionate has a half-life of up to 8 days because of its eight-carbon atom ester chain, compared with 4 to 8 days for testosterone enanthate which has a carboxylic acid ester, enanthoic acid composed of seven carbon atoms. All esters are hepatically metabolized by the Cytochrome P450.

Peak serum concentrations are achieved within 72 h, followed by an exponential decay. Many men describe a testosterone crash toward the end of the cycle. Nadir levels are useful to adjust the frequency and dose on an individual basis. Patients taking injectable testosterone are more susceptible to erythrocytosis. One study found an increase in Hct in 24% of patients after injections of testosterone cypionate without any adverse effects. Older patients are much more likely to develop erythrocytosis, and caution should be taken in this population.

Subcutaneous pellets Testopel
General principles
- Testopel provides adequate levels of testosterone for at least 3 months
- Current FDA-approved dosing schedules are based on anachronistic label without pharmacokinetic backup resulting in underdosing (see **Table 4**)
- Convenience of not having a daily application but the inconvenience of a quarterly office visit for a surgical procedure
- Repeated insertions cause scarring, leading to insertional pain, hematomas and extrusions.

- Levels are tested at the nadir, shortly before re-insertion, to give dosage adjustment
- Package insert restricts flexible dosing

SC 75 mg crystalline testosterone pellets have been available for decades having been FDA approved in 1972 (Bartor Phamacal) and re-introduced into the commercial market in 2008 (Testopel, Slate Pharmaceuticals). Testopel pellets are currently the only long-acting FDA-approved pellet available in the United States. No pharmacokinetic studies were done prior to approval in 1972. Recommended dosing was based on levels achieved with testosterone propionate, an esterified testosterone no longer marketed, with a half-life of 4.5 days. The recommended doing is 4 to 6 pellets (300–450) every 3 to 6 months. That would translate to a maximum and minimum dose of 37.5 mg/wk (6 pellets every 3 months) and 9 mg/wk (4 pellets every 6 months), respectively. Even the testosterone ester with the longest half-life, testosterone undecanoate, is dosed every 10 weeks at a dose of 750 mg (75 mg a week). The current recommended dosing schedule realistically results in subtherapeutic dosing and exposes patients to more frequent pellet insertions.[47] In a multi-institutional retrospective study, Testopel provided sustained levels of testosterone for at least 4 months in men with testosterone deficiency. Implantation of more than 8 pellets achieved optimal results with respect to peak mean testosterone level and duration of effect. Ninety-five percent of men received at least 10 pellets (750 mgs).

Testosterone pellets were generally well tolerated. Retrospective pharmacokinetic studies with Testopel have shown that men with a body mass index (BMI) greater than 25 attained lower total testosterone peaks with slower decay than men with BMI less than 25. No differences were seen in decay rates for men with multiple implant rounds, and no differences in testosterone peaks or decay rates were seen in men with preimplantation testosterone level less than 300 or greater than or equal to 300 ng/dL. They reported that the levels were not impacted by the number of insertions.[48] Anecdotally, as the number of insertions increase, and the SC tissues scar from repeated insertions there is a tendency for more insertional pain, hematomas, and extrusions. There is no guidance provided as to the timing of checking the levels, but it would seem logical to test at the nadir, shortly before re-insertion to adjust the number of pellets and the frequency of insertion.

The pellets typically dissolve more than 4 to 6 months and thus do not need to be removed. Potential benefits of Testopel include a lack of

Table 5
Testosterone therapies

Formulation	Mode of Delivery	Dose	Starting Dose	Application Site
Topical				
Androgel® 1% (Testosterone Gel)	Packet Pump	25 mg/2.5 g 50 mg/5 g	50 mg of testosterone once daily in the AM 2 pumps on each shoulder	Shoulders/upper arms and/or abdomen Shoulders and/or upper arms
Androgel® 1.62% (Testosterone Gel)	Packet Pump	12.5 mg/actuation 20.25 m	40.5 mg testosterone daily in the AM	Shoulders and/or upper arms
Testim® 1% (Testosterone Gel)	Tube Pump	40.5 mg 20.25 mg testosterone per actuation.	1 pump on each shoulder 50 mg daily in the AM	Shoulders and/or upper arms Inner or front of thighs
Fortesta® 2% (Testosterone Gel)	Tube, Packet	5 and 10 g tubes which contain 50 and 100 mg of testosterone, respectively. 10 mg/actuation	2 pumps each thigh daily in the AM	Shoulders and/or upper arms
Vogelxo® (Testosterone Gel)	Pump	50 mg of testosterone in a unit-dose tube, 50 mg in a unit-dose packet, 12.5 mg per actuation	50 mg of testosterone daily at the same time 4 pumps	Shoulders and/or upper arms
Transdermal Androderm®	Patch	2 mg/d, 2.5 mg/d, 4 mg/d and 5 mg/d	One 4 mg/d patches applied at night (10 PM)	Back, abdomen, upper arms, or thighs
Intranasal Gel Natesto®	Pump	5.5 mg of testosterone/pump actuation	11 mg of testosterone (2 pump actuations, one per nostril) three times daily (6–8 h apart)	Intranasal
Oral JATENZO® (Testosterone Undecanoate)	Capsule	158 mg, 198 mg, 237 mg	237 mg once in the morning and once in the evening	Oral
Pellet Testopel®	Pellet	75 mg/pellet	150–450 mg every 3–6 mo	Subcutaneous; Subdermal fat of the buttocks, lower abdominal wall, or thigh
Intramuscular Injection Testosterone Cypionate, Enanthate AVEED®	Solution Solution	100 mg/mL 10 mL vial; 200 mg/mL 1- or 10-mL vial 750 mg/3 mL (250 mg/mL)	75–100 mg once weekly or 150–200 mg every 2 wk [19] 3 mL (750 mg) at initiation at 4 wk, and every 10 wk thereafter	Intramuscular-Gluteal muscle or lateral upper thigh Gluteal muscle
Subcutaneous XYOSTED®	Solution in Autoinjector	50 mg/0.5 mL; 75 mg/0.5 mL; 100 mg/0.5 mL	75 mg subcutaneously once weekly	Subcutaneously in the abdominal region

transference and assurance on the part of the provider that the patient has received his treatment. There is the convenience of not having a daily application but the inconvenience of a quarterly office visit at the mercy of the provider's schedule. Potential risks of Testopel are bleeding, infection, expulsion of the pellets, pain, and bruising. The infections and extrusion rates were reported at 1.1% and 0.4%, respectively.[48]

The pellets are placed SC with a 2 mm anesthetized incision through a proprietary trocar in the gluteal fat pad. The procedure usually takes 10 min of the provider's time. Patients are then observed for an additional 10 min thereafter, applying pressure to the insertion site. In all, between the patient registration, the procedure and post insertion observation and follow-up scheduling, approximately 30 min of office time are needed. Medicare will reimburse for no more than six pellets every 3 months at invoice costs minus a mandated withhold of 6% because of the Budget Reconciliation Act. As the procedure is scheduled, only the insertion code (11980) is allowed without an evaluation and management (E/M) office visit code. With an individual pellet cost of approximately $100 each and the Medicare reimbursement for the insertion of $94, an uncomplicated 30-min office visit will result in a $60 payment, be repeated 4 times a year and take the space of four new patient visits or 8 established patients. Though some third-party payers may reimburse the above invoice cost and pay more for the insertion, the time commitment is the same. This is not a sustainable model for practice growth regardless of the payer.

Subcutaneous injections (Xyosted)
General principles
- Generic testosterone enanthate in an expensive proprietary injector
- Convenient, well tolerated, and easily administered
- Poorly reimbursed by insurance companies
- Excellent pharmacokinetics
- Validates the concept of SC testosterone enanthate
- Poor insurance coverage

The parenteral administration of testosterone has historically been intramuscular. The package insert for both generic testosterone cypionate and testosterone enanthate specifically mentions intramuscular injections. Recently SC injections have become increasingly popular. Theoretically, SC deposition of testosterone esters in the relatively hypovascular subdermal space results in a more stable, slower absorption from the lymphatic

and vascular spaces and unlike IM injections is less subject to muscular contraction[49] In a study of 64 female-to-male transgender patients normal male levels were achieved in all patient with weekly SC injections of TE or TC and were preferred to IM injections.[49,50] The use of weekly SC testosterone enanthate with a proprietary injector, Xyosted, was approved by the FDA in 2018. TE has a half-life of approximately 4 to 7 days.[51] Xyosted comes in 50, 75, and 100 mg single-dose syringes, assembled in a pressure-assisted autoinjector for SC administration. During a 52-week follow-up period, upward dose titration based on levels only was necessary for up to 30% of the men on 50 mg at week 6,11% on men on 75 mg at week 6 and none on 100 mg at week 6. Downward titration occurred in 11% of men on 75 mg at week 6 and up to 45% on 100 mg at week 6. Blinded dose adjustments if needed were based on nadir levels independent of symptoms at weeks 6 7, 13, 19, 27, and 39. The age range tested was 18 to 75 with BMI <40. The patient reported ease of use was uniformly high and 95% of patients reported no injection-related pain. Therapeutic levels (300–1000 ng/dL) were achieved in 92.7% of patients. Whereas slightly less than 10% of patients achieved a level of greater than 1500 ng/dL, none surpassed 1800 ng/dL.[52] Increases in Hct to ≥55% were reported for 12 of the 283 patients in the 2 clinical studies, representing 4.2% of patients who received Xyosted for up to 1 year.

Long-acting testosterone AVEED
General principles
- Long-acting testosterone is dispensed in castor oil with enhances its ability to release over time
- Injected every 10 weeks requiring a 30-min office visit
- Rare cases of spontaneous POME have been reported as adverse event per-injection rate of <1%
- Patients are required to remain in the doctor's office for 30 min after their dose to observe for POME
- Package insert limits the flexibility of dosing schedule and amounts

AVEED is the only long-acting testosterone injection on the US market. AVEED contains 750 mg of TU, which is injected IM in 3 mL of castor oil. TU is injected with a castor oil carrier, which enhances its ability to release slowly over time. The first injection with AVEED requires a 4-week repeat injection. Following this initial repeat injection, AVEED is injected every 10 weeks. There is no allowance for adjusting the dosing schedule based on levels. As there is only one dose and one dosing schedule on the FDA label, individualization of the regimen is difficult to obtain from third-party payers. The most common adverse events associated with AVEED include acne and pain at the injection site. Rare cases of pulmonary oil micro embolism (POME) have been reported. In a 4.3-year post-marketing review of their Endo Pharmaceuticals Inc safety database, with 90,092 doses, 28 of 633 individual case safety reports were classified as POME, for a yearly spontaneously reported adverse event per-injection rate of less than 1%. Twenty one of the 22 for which the outcome was reported, resolved, and of those with a resolution time reported, most (13 of 17) resolved in 30 min. One fatality was reported 18 months after a documented POME event and appeared unrelated to the reported testosterone undecanoate injection. Despite the POME event, 64% of patients continued the testosterone undecanoate. As part of the AVEED Risk Evaluation and Mitigation Strategy Program[53] patients are required to remain in the doctor's office for 30 min and be observed for POME. Continuation of therapy should be based on achieving symptom resolution for the treatment period. Nadir levels should be checked. If symptomatic improvement is not obtained and eugonadal levels are not maintained throughout the 10-week period, consideration should be given to an alternative replacement modality.

SUMMARY

There is a vast abundance of therapeutic modalities for hypogonadism, each with its own mode of delivery, pharmacokinetic profile, dosing sequence, and side effect profile leading to various advantages and disadvantages. It is important to understand the physiology of hypogonadism and the pharmacokinetics of each testosterone formulation to be able to make the right choice for the patient. Factors contributing to adherence of therapy include patient expectations, follow-up, knowledge about each formulation, access, cost, insurance coverage, and east of use. The practitioner is best using the modality with which he/she is most familiar. Careful consideration of the needs of the patient is important. Continuation of therapy should be predicated on achieving amelioration of hypogonadal symptoms, achieving therapeutic levels in a compliant patient.

DISCLOSURE

No conflict of interests.

REFERENCES

1. Basaria SWJ, Dobbs AS. Anabolic-Androgenic Steroid Therapy in the treatment of chronic diseases. J Clin Endocrinol Metab 2001;86(11):5108–17.
2. Dunn JF, Nisula BC, Rodbard D. Transport of steroid hormones: binding of 21 endogenous steroids to both testosterone-binding globulin and corticosteroid-binding globulin in human plasma. J Clin Endocrinol Metab 1981;53(1):58–68.
3. Bhasin S, Cunningham GR, Hayes FJ, et al. Testosterone therapy in men with androgen deficiency syndromes: an Endocrine Society clinical practice guideline. J Clin Endocrinol Metab 2010;95(6):2536–59.
4. Basaria S. Male hypogonadism. Lancet 2014;5–11.
5. Melmed S, Polonsky KS, Reed LP, et al. Williams textbook of endocrinology. Elsevier Health Sciences; 2015.
6. White C, MJ F-B, NM M, et al. The pharmacokinetics of intravenous testosterone in elderly men with coronary artery disease. J Clin Pharmacol 1998;38(9):792–7.
7. Oettel M. Testosterone metabolism,dose-response relationships and receptor polymorphisms:selected pharmacologi.toxicological considerations on benefits versus the risks of testosterone therpay in men. Aging Male 2003;6(4):230–56.
8. Bhasin SWL, Casaburi R, Singh AB, et al. Testosterone doe-response relationships in healthy young men. Am J Physiol Endocrinol Metab 2001;281:E1172–81.
9. Simoncini TGA. Non-genomic actions of sex steroid hormones. Eur J Endocrtinology 2003;148:281–92.
10. Papakonstanti EAKM, Castanas E, Stounaras C. A rapid,nongenomic,signnaling pathway regulates the actin reorganization induced by activation of membrane testosterone receptors. Mol Endocrinol 2003;17:870–81.
11. Heinlein CACC. The roles of androgen receptors and androgen-binding proteions in non genomic androgen action. Mol Endocrinol 2002;16:2181–7.
12. Brambilla DJ, O'Donnell AB, Matsumoto AM, et al. Intraindividual variation in levels of serum testosterone and other reproductive and adrenal hormones in men. Clin Endocrinol (Oxf) 2007;67(6):853–62.
13. Brambilla DJ, Matsumoto AM, Araujo AB, et al. The effect of diurnal variation on clinical measurement of serum testosterone and other sex hormone levels in men. J Clin Endocrinol Metab 2009;94(3):907–13.
14. Gonzalez-Sales M, Barriere O, Tremblay PO, et al. Modeling Testosterone Circadian Rhythm in Hypogonadal Males: Effect of Age and Circannual Variations. AAPS J 2016;18(1):217–27.
15. Welliver RC Jr, Wiser HJ, Brannigan RE, et al. Validity of midday total testosterone levels in older men with erectile dysfunction. J Urol 2014;192(1):165–9.

16. Garnick MB. Testosterone replacement therapy faces FDA scrutiny. JAMA 2015;313(6):563–4.

17. Caronia LM, Dwyer AA, Hayden D, et al. Abrupt decrease in serum testosterone levels after an oral glucose load in men: implications for screening for hypogonadism. Clin Endocrinol (Oxf) 2013;78(2): 291–6.

18. Lehtihet M, Arver S, Bartuseviciene I, et al. S-testosterone decrease after a mixed meal in healthy men independent of SHBG and gonadotrophin levels. Andrologia 2012;44(6):405–10.

19. Mulhall JP, Trost LW, Brannigan RE, et al. Evaluation and management of testosterone deficiency: AUA guideline. J Urol 2018;200(2):423–32.

20. Locke JA, Flannigan R, Gunther OP, et al. Testosterone therapy: Prescribing and monitoring patterns of practice in British Columbia. Can Urol Assoc J 2021;15(2):E110–7.

21. Grabner M, Hepp Z, Raval A, et al. Topical testosterone therapy adherence and outcomes among men with primary or secondary hypogonadism. J Sex Med 2018;15(2):148–58.

22. Schoenfeld MJ, Shortridge E, Cui Z, et al. Medication adherence and treatment patterns for hypogonadal patients treated with topical testosterone therapy: a retrospective medical claims analysis. J Sex Med 2013;10(5):1401–9.

23. Donatucci C, Cui Z, Fang Y, et al. Long-term treatment patterns of testosterone replacement medications. J Sex Med 2014;11(8):2092–9.

24. Straftis AA, Gray PB. Sex, Energy, Well-Being and Low Testosterone: An Exploratory Survey of U.S. Men's Experiences on Prescription Testosterone. Int J Environ Res Public Health 2019;16(18). https://doi.org/10.3390/ijerph16183261.

25. Gilbert K, Cimmino CB, Beebe LC, et al. Gaps in patient knowledge about risks and benefits of testosterone replacement therapy. Urology 2017;103: 27–33.

26. Dwyer AA, Tiemensma J, Quinton R, et al. Adherence to treatment in men with hypogonadotrophic hypogonadism. Clin Endocrinol (Oxf) 2017;86(3): 377–83.

27. Shoskes JJ, Wilson MK, Spinner ML. Pharmacology of testosterone replacement therapy preparations. Transl Androl Urol 2016;5(6):834–43.

28. Swerdloff RS, Wang C, Cunningham G, et al. Long-term pharmacokinetics of transdermal testosterone gel in hypogonadal men. J Clin Endocrinol Metab 2000;85(12):4500–10.

29. Miller J, Britto M, Fitzpatrick S, et al. Pharmacokinetics and relative bioavailability of absorbed testosterone after administration of a 1.62% testosterone gel to different application sites in men with hypogonadism. Endocr Pract 2011;17(4):574–83.

30. Hadgraft J, Lane ME. Transdermal delivery of testosterone. Eur J Pharm Biopharm 2015;92:42–8.

31. McNicholas T, Ong T. Review of testim gel. Expert Opin Pharmacother 2006;7(4):477–84.

32. Dobs AS, McGettigan J, Norwood P, et al. A novel testosterone 2% gel for the treatment of hypogonadal males. J Androl 2012;33(4):601–7. https://doi.org/10.2164/jandrol.111.014308.

33. Morgentaler A, McGettigan J, Xiang Q, et al. Pharmacokinetics and drying time of testosterone 2% gel in men with hypogonadism: a multicenter, open-label, single-arm trial. Int J Impot Res 2015; 27(2):41–5.

34. Dobs AS, Meikle AW, Arver S, et al. Pharmacokinetics, efficacy, and safety of a permeation-enhanced testosterone transdermal system in comparison with bi-weekly injections of testosterone enanthate for the treatment of hypogonadal men. J Clin Endocrinol Metab 1999;84(10):3469–78.

35. Available at: https://www.accessdata.fda.gov/drugsatfda_docs/label/2011/020489s025lbl.pdf.

36. Mattern C, Hoffmann C, Morley JE, et al. Testosterone supplementation for hypogonadal men by the nasal route. Aging Male 2008;11(4):171–8. https://doi.org/10.1080/13685530802351974.

37. Banks WA, Morley JE, Niehoff ML, et al. Delivery of testosterone to the brain by intranasal administration: comparison to intravenous testosterone. J Drug Target 2009;17(2):91–7.

38. Rogol AD, Tkachenko N, Bryson N. Natesto , a novel testosterone nasal gel, normalizes androgen levels in hypogonadal men. Andrology 2016;4(1): 46–54.

39. Masterson T, Molina M, Ibrahim E, et al. Natesto effects on reproductive hormones and semen parameters: results from an ongoing single-center, investigator-initiated phase IV clinical trial. Eur Urol Focus 2018;4(3):333–5.

40. Available at: https://www.accessdata.fda.gov/drugsatfda_docs/label/2014/205488s000lbl.pdf.

41. Sclar DA, Tartaglione TA, Fine MJ. Overview of issues related to medical compliance with implications for the outpatient management of infectious diseases. Infect Agents Dis 1994;3(5):266–73.

42. Nieschlag E, Mauss J, Coert A, et al. Plasma androgen levels in men after oral administration of testosterone or testosterone undecanoate. Acta Endocrinol (Copenh) 1975;79(2):366–74.

43. Horst HJ, Holtje WJ, Dennis M, et al. Lymphatic absorption and metabolism of orally administered testosterone undecanoate in man. Klin Wochenschr 1976;54(18):875–9.

44. Swerdloff RS, Dudley RE. A new oral testosterone undecanoate therapy comes of age for the treatment of hypogonadal men. Ther Adv Urol 2020;12. 1756287220937232.

45. Schurmeyer T, Wickings EJ, Freischem CW, et al. Saliva and serum testosterone following oral testosterone undecanoate administration in normal and

hypogonadal men. Acta Endocrinol (Copenh) 1983; 102(3):456–62.

46. Bagchus WM, Hust R, Maris F, et al. Important effect of food on the bioavailability of oral testosterone undecanoate. Pharmacotherapy 2003;23(3):319–25.

47. McCullough A. A Review of Testosterone Pellets in the Treatment of Hypogonadism. Curr Sex Health Rep 2014;6(4):265–9.

48. Pastuszak AW, Mittakanti H, Liu JS, et al. Pharmacokinetic evaluation and dosing of subcutaneous testosterone pellets. J Androl 2012;33(5):927–37.

49. Figueiredo MG, Gagliano-Juca T, Basaria S. Testosterone Therapy with Subcutaneous Injections: A Safe, Practical and Reasonable Option. J Clin Endocrinol Metab 2021. https://doi.org/10.1210/clinem/dgab772.

50. Spratt DI, Stewart II, Savage C, et al. Subcutaneous injection of testosterone is an effective and preferred alternative to intramuscular injection: demonstration in female-to-male transgender patients. J Clin Endocrinol Metab 2017;102(7):2349–55.

51. Rohayem J, Tüttelmann F, Nieschlag E, et al. Hypothalamisch bedingter hypogonadotroper Hypogonadismus. In: Nieschlag E, Behre HM, Kliesch S, et al, editors. Andrologie: grundlagen und Klinik der reproduktiven Gesundheit des Mannes. Berlin Heidelberg: Springer; 2020. p. 1–10.

52. Kaminetsky JC, McCullough A, Hwang K, et al. A 52-week study of dose adjusted subcutaneous testosterone enanthate in oil self-administered via disposable auto-injector. J Urol 2019;201(3):587–94.

53. Pastuszak AW, Hu Y, Freid JD. Occurrence of pulmonary oil microembolism after testosterone undecanoate injection: a postmarketing safety analysis. Sex Med 2020;8(2):237–42.

The Prostate as an Endocrine Organ
Its Modulation of Serum Testosterone

Kevin R. Loughlin, MD, MBA

KEYWORDS

- Prostate cancer • Benign prostatic hypertrophy • Testosterone • Dihydrotestosterone • LH • FSH
- Inhibin

KEY POINTS

- Provocative findings suggest that the prostate gland may have more endocrine functions than previously appreciated.
- Prostate cancer, but not benign prostatic hyperplasia, appears to exert some modulation of the hypothalamic-pituitary axis.
- The increase of serum testosterone following a radical prostatectomy seems to be, at least, in part influenced by a factor or factors produced by prostate cancer.
- Inhibin and dihydrotestosterone have been proposed as possible substances elaborated by prostate cancer that influence the hypothalamic-pituitary axis and thereby modulate postprostatectomy serum testosterone levels.

INTRODUCTION

Aside from nonmelanoma skin cancer, prostate cancer is the most common cancer among men in the United States,[1] and benign prostatic hyperplasia (BPH) is the most common benign tumor found in men.[2] Until recently, its endocrine functions and possible influence on the hypothalamic-pituitary axis have been relatively understudied. This review summarizes the current understanding of the potential endocrine functions of prostate cancer and benign prostate tissue.

Emerging Observations

In 1998, Miller and colleagues[3] reported on 63 men, ages 43 to 67 years, who had a phlebotomy performed immediately before and one year following a radical retropubic prostatectomy. Serum testosterone, percent-free testosterone, dihydrotestosterone (DHT), estradiol, luteinizing hormone (LH), follicle-stimulating hormone (FSH), serum hormone–binding globulin (SHBG), and prolactin were measured. They reported that following radical prostatectomy there was a statistically significant increase in serum testosterone, free testosterone, estradiol, LH, and FSH ($p < 0.0001$) and a decrease in serum DHT ($p < 0.0001$). There was no statistically significant correlation between any serum hormone and sample storage time, patient age, or prostate volume. In addition, serum hormone changes did not correlate with pathological stage or histological grade for these patients. The investigators postulated that DHT and inhibin were 2 known factors produced by the prostate that could induce this effect.

In 2002, Madersbacher and colleagues[4] followed the Hopkins study with a diverse group of patients, 49 underwent a radical prostatectomy for prostate cancer, 51 underwent a transurethral resection of the prostate (TURP) for BPH, and 46 were managed conservatively for lower urinary tract symptoms. Serum levels of testosterone, LH, and FSH were measured at baseline and 6 and 12 months later in all patients.

There were no significant endocrine changes observed in the observation or TURP groups at 6

Vascular Biology Research Laboratory, Boston Children's Hospital, Harvard Medical School, Boston, MA 02114, USA
E-mail address: kloughlin@partners.org

Urol Clin N Am 49 (2022) 695–697
https://doi.org/10.1016/j.ucl.2022.07.001
0094-0143/22/

and 12 months after baseline. However, in contrast, in the prostate cancer group followed after radical prostatectomy, the LH increased from 5.2 to 8.9 mIU/mL (p = 0.0004) and the FSH increased from 5.7 to 9.3 mIU/mL (p = 0.0003) 12 months after radical prostatectomy (p = 0.0003). The increase of total testosterone from 3.9 to 4.4 ng/mL did not reach statistical significance (p = 0.18). At 12 months after radical prostatectomy, no changes from baseline were observed in patients with a Gleason score of 2 to 6, but in those patients with a Gleason score of 7 to 10, the serum testosterone more than doubled. However, the LH and FSH levels were comparable in both low- and high-grade tumors at 12 months.

The investigators concluded from this study that prostate cancer and not benign prostate tissue mediated the changes in the hypothalamic-pituitary axis and that the changes were more pronounced in the higher grade tumors.

In 2010, Olsson and colleagues[5] examined the serum levels of testosterone, DHT, SHBG, LH, and FSH in 53 patients before and 90 days after radical prostatectomy. Inhibin B levels were analyzed before and 90 days postoperatively in 44 patients.

LH levels increased from 3.24 ± 0.32 mIU/mL to 4.97 mIU/mL ± 0.48 (p = 0.0001), and FSH levels increased from 6.62 ± 0.88 to 8.04 ± 1.1 mIU/mL (p = 0.0001), and DHT decreased from 482 ± 39.7 pg/mL to 419 ± 35.7 pg/mL (p = 0.028).

However, there were no significant changes in preoperative and postoperative levels in testosterone, free testosterone, or SHBG. Of additional importance was the finding that the inhibin B levels were unchanged from preoperative to postoperative levels (166.3 ± 13.5 vs 167.7 ± 12.1 ng/mL). These investigators also observed that the Gleason score was not correlated with the baseline serum androgen levels or changes in the androgen levels 3 months after the radical prostatectomy.

In 2013 Gacci and colleagues[6] studied 100 patients with clinically localized prostate cancer who were treated with a radical retropubic prostatectomy. Serum levels of testosterone, LH, and FSH were measured at baseline and 1 and 3 months postoperatively.

At 1 month after radical prostatectomy, serum testosterone levels were decreased from 15.3 to 13.8 nmol/L (p = 0.021), however, by 3 months the testosterone level had increased to 14.4 nmol/L (p = 0.372). In contrast the log LH level was increased at 1 and 3 months postsurgery compared with the baseline (baseline vs 1 month log LH 0.54 vs 0.68 mIU/mL p < 0.0001), and at 3 months it remained elevated with log LH 0.54 versus 0.65 mIU/mL (p < 0.0001).

Similarly, the postsurgery FSH levels were elevated. At 1 month, the log FSH level increased from 0.74 to 0.80 mIU/mL (p = 0.0001) and remained elevated at 3 months log FSH (0.74 to 0.82 mIU/mL; p < 0.0001).

The investigators interpreted their results as suggesting that the testosterone was transiently decreased at 1 month after radical prostatectomy and the elevated LH observed at 1 month persisted. The serum T had returned to almost preoperative T levels with a persistent LH elevation, which was consistent with a compensated hypergonadotropic hypogonadism 3 months after radical prostatectomy.

The Putative Role of Inhibin

It would appear that the prostate elaborates a factor or factors that interact with the hypothalamic-pituitary axis and thereby influences postprostatectomy testosterone levels. Walsh has speculated that this substance might be inhibin.[7]

Inhibin A and B are 2 glycoproteins that are secreted by Sertoli cells in the testes and granulosa cells in the ovaries and inhibit FSH by direct action on the pituitary.[8] Risbridger and colleagues[9] demonstrated an elevated expression of inhibin alpha in prostate cancer. In addition to its role in the reproductive tract of men and women, Balanathan and colleagues[10] have demonstrated the inhibin alpha subunit to be pro-tumorigenic and prometastatic and is associated with extracapsular spread in advanced prostate cancer.

However, as mentioned earlier, although Olsson and colleagues[5] found a 53% increase in serum LH and a 21% increase in serum FSH and a 13% decrease in DHT following radical prostatectomy, they found the serum inhibin B levels were unchanged postoperatively from preoperative levels.

Additional study regarding the possible relationship between inhibin and the low testosterone levels in patients with hypogonadal prostate cancer was provided by Lackner and colleagues.[11] They entered 126 men with prostate cancer and 70 men with BPH in their study. The serum inhibin levels did not differ significantly between the patients with BPH and those with prostate cancer (150.0 vs 131.75 pg/mL, p = 0.062), between those with hypogonadal and eugonadal disease (143.0 vs 146.5 pg/mL, p = 0.573), or those with low-grade and high-grade cancer (151.5 vs 146.0 pg/mL, p = 0.830). Men with higher grade cancer had lower levels of serum testosterone than did those with low-grade cancer (3.49 vs 4.09, p = 0.056).

Future Directions

There are several intriguing questions regarding prostate cancer and serum testosterone:

1. Do the serum T and the gonadotropins change over time postoperatively and does recurrent prostate cancer interfere with the hypothalamic-pituitary axis? If so, could a delayed but gradual decrease in serum testosterone herald recurrent prostate cancer and function as a surrogate biomarker?
2. Will further studies confirm the initial observations that malignant, but not benign, prostate tissue mediates the observed effect on serum testosterone?
3. If prostate cancer is the mediator of the observed changes in serum testosterone, does a higher grade cancer cause a more profound depression?
4. If subsequent studies confirm that inhibin is not the vehicle for the observed changes in testosterone, then what substance or substances are the mediators?

SUMMARY

For many years there has been an ongoing controversy regarding the influence of serum testosterone levels and the development of prostate cancer. In 2015, the author and his colleagues reported a literature review that confirmed this controversy. They identified 45 studies that examined this relationship and 18 found a relationship between prostate cancer and low testosterone, 17 reported a relationship with high serum testosterone, and 10 found no relationship between the serum testosterone level and prostate cancer.[12]

Walsh and his group made the observation that prostate cancer influenced testosterone level almost a quarter of a century ago. For most of the subsequent years, that observation has gone largely ignored and underinvestigated. There has been a plethora of articles reporting conflicting results examining the hypothesis that serum testosterone influences the development of prostate cancer. It is long overdue to begin looking in the opposite direction that it may be the prostate cancer that influences the serum testosterone and not the other way around.

REFERENCES

1. Prostate Cancer Statistics. Available at: Cdc.gov/cancer/prostate/statistics/index.html. Accessed January 20, 2022.
2. Benign Prostatic Hyperplasia(BPH) Johns Hopkins Medicine-Health. Available at: https://www.hopkinsmedicine.org/health/conditions-and-disease/benign-prostatic-hyperplasia-bph. Accessed January 20, 2022.
3. Miller LR, Partin AW, Chen DW, et al. Influence of radical prostatectomy on serum hormone levels. J Urol 1998;160:449–53.
4. Madersbacher S, Schatzl G, Bieglmayer C, et al. Impact of radical prostatectomy and TURP on the hypothalamic-pituitary-gonadal hormone axis. Urology 2002;60(5):869–74.
5. Olsson M, Ekstrom L, Schulze J, et al. Radical prostatectomy: influence on serum and urinary androgen levels. Prostate 2010;70:200–5.
6. Gacci M, Tosi N, Vittori G, et al. Changes in sex hormone levels after radical prostatectomy: Results of a longitudinal cohort study. Oncol Lett 2013;6(2):529–33.
7. Walsh PC. Editorial comment: impact of radical prostatectomy and TURP on the hypothalamic-pituitary-gonadal hormone axis. J.Urol. 2003;170:319–20.
8. Franchimont P, Hazee-Hagelstein MT, Jaspar M, et al. Inhibin and related peptides. Mechanisms of action and regulation of secretion. J Steroid Biochem 1989;32(1B):193–7.
9. Risbridger GP, Shibata A, Ferguson KL, et al. Elevated expression of inhibin alpha in prostate cancer. J Urol 2004;171:192–6.
10. Balanathan P, Williams ED, Wang H, et al. Elevated level of inhibin alpha subunit is pro-tumourigenic and pro-metastatic and associated with extracapsular spread in advanced prostate cancer. Br J Cancer 2009;100(11):1784–93.
11. Lackner JE, Maerk I, Keller A, et al. Serum inhibin-not a cause of low testosterone levels in hypogonadal prostate cancer? Urology 2008;72(5):1121–4.
12. Klap J, Schmid M, Loughlin KR. The relationship between total testosterone levels and prostate cancer: a review of the continuing controversy. J.Urol. 2015;193(2):403–13.

UNITED STATES POSTAL SERVICE ®
Statement of Ownership, Management, and Circulation
(All Periodicals Publications Except Requester Publications)

1. Publication Title	2. Publication Number	3. Filing Date
UROLOGIC CLINICS OF NORTH AMERICA	000 – 711	9/18/2022

4. Issue Frequency	5. Number of Issues Published Annually	6. Annual Subscription Price
FEB, MAY, AUG, NOV	4	$403.00

7. Complete Mailing Address of Known Office of Publication (Not printer) (Street, city, county, state, and ZIP+4®)

ELSEVIER INC.
230 Park Avenue, Suite 800
New York, NY 10169

Contact Person: Malathi Samayan
Telephone (Include area code): 91-44-4299-4507

8. Complete Mailing Address of Headquarters or General Business Office of Publisher (Not printer)

ELSEVIER INC.
230 Park Avenue, Suite 800
New York, NY 10169

9. Full Names and Complete Mailing Addresses of Publisher, Editor, and Managing Editor (Do not leave blank)

Publisher (Name and complete mailing address)

Dolores Meloni, ELSEVIER INC.
1600 JOHN F KENNEDY BLVD, SUITE 1800
PHILADELPHIA, PA 19103-2899

Editor (Name and complete mailing address)

KERRY HOLLAND, ELSEVIER INC.
1600 JOHN F KENNEDY BLVD, SUITE 1800
PHILADELPHIA, PA 19103-2899

Managing Editor (Name and complete mailing address)

PATRICK MANLEY, ELSEVIER INC.
1600 JOHN F KENNEDY BLVD, SUITE 1800
PHILADELPHIA, PA 19103-2899

10. Owner (Do not leave blank. If the publication is owned by a corporation, give the name and address of the corporation immediately followed by the names and addresses of all stockholders owning or holding 1 percent or more of the total amount of stock. If not owned by a corporation, give the names and addresses of the individual owners. If owned by a partnership or other unincorporated firm, give its name and address as well as those of each individual owner. If the publication is published by a nonprofit organization, give its name and address.)

Full Name	Complete Mailing Address
WHOLLY OWNED SUBSIDIARY OF REED/ELSEVIER, US HOLDINGS	1600 JOHN F KENNEDY BLVD, SUITE 1800 PHILADELPHIA, PA 19103-2899

11. Known Bondholders, Mortgagees, and Other Security Holders Owning or Holding 1 Percent or More of Total Amount of Bonds, Mortgages, or Other Securities. If none, check box ▶ ☐ None

Full Name	Complete Mailing Address
N/A	

12. Tax Status (For completion by nonprofit organizations authorized to mail at nonprofit rates) (Check one)
The purpose, function, and nonprofit status of this organization and the exempt status for federal income tax purposes:
☒ Has Not Changed During Preceding 12 Months
☐ Has Changed During Preceding 12 Months (Publisher must submit explanation of change with this statement)

PS Form 3526, July 2014 [Page 1 of 4 (see instructions page 4)] PSN: 7530-01-000-9931   PRIVACY NOTICE: See our privacy policy on www.usps.com.

13. Publication Title	14. Issue Date for Circulation Data Below
UROLOGIC CLINICS OF NORTH AMERICA	MAY 2022

15. Extent and Nature of Circulation			Average No. Copies Each Issue During Preceding 12 Months	No. Copies of Single Issue Published Nearest to Filing Date
a. Total Number of Copies (Net press run)			310	259
b. Paid Circulation (By Mail and Outside the Mail)	(1)	Mailed Outside-County Paid Subscriptions Stated on PS Form 3541 (Include paid distribution above nominal rate, advertiser's proof copies, and exchange copies)	147	117
	(2)	Mailed In-County Paid Subscriptions Stated on PS Form 3541 (Include paid distribution above nominal rate, advertiser's proof copies, and exchange copies)	0	0
	(3)	Paid Distribution Outside the Mails Including Sales Through Dealers and Carriers, Street Vendors, Counter Sales, and Other Paid Distribution Outside USPS®	113	80
	(4)	Paid Distribution by Other Classes of Mail Through the USPS (e.g. First-Class Mail®)	0	0
c. Total Paid Distribution (Sum of 15b (1), (2), (3), and (4)) ▶			260	197
d. Free or Nominal Rate Distribution (By Mail and Outside the Mail)	(1)	Free or Nominal Rate Outside-County Copies included on PS Form 3541	34	46
	(2)	Free or Nominal Rate In-County Copies included on PS Form 3541	0	0
	(3)	Free or Nominal Rate Copies Mailed at Other Classes Through the USPS (e.g. First-Class Mail)	0	0
	(4)	Free or Nominal Rate Distribution Outside the Mail (Carriers or other means)	0	0
e. Total Free or Nominal Rate Distribution (Sum of 15d (1), (2), (3) and (4)) ▶			34	46
f. Total Distribution (Sum of 15c and 15e) ▶			294	243
g. Copies not Distributed (See Instructions to Publishers #4 (page #3)) ▶			16	16
h. Total (Sum of 15f and g) ▶			310	259
i. Percent Paid (15c divided by 15f times 100) ▶			88.43%	81.06%

* If you are claiming electronic copies, go to line 16 on page 3. If you are not claiming electronic copies, skip to line 17 on page 3.

PS Form 3526, July 2014 (Page 2 of 4)

16. Electronic Copy Circulation		Average No. Copies Each Issue During Preceding 12 Months	No. Copies of Single Issue Published Nearest to Filing Date
a. Paid Electronic Copies ▶			
b. Total Paid Print Copies (Line 15c) + Paid Electronic Copies (Line 16a) ▶			
c. Total Print Distribution (Line 15f) + Paid Electronic Copies (Line 16a) ▶			
d. Percent Paid (Both Print & Electronic Copies) (16b divided by 16c × 100) ▶			

☒ I certify that 50% of all my distributed copies (electronic and print) are paid above a nominal price.

17. Publication of Statement of Ownership

☒ If the publication is a general publication, publication of this statement is required. Will be printed
in the NOVEMBER 2022 issue of this publication.   ☐ Publication not required.

18. Signature and Title of Editor, Publisher, Business Manager, or Owner

Malathi Samayan - Distribution Controller   *Malathi Samayan*   Date 9/18/2022

I certify that all information furnished on this form is true and complete. I understand that anyone who furnishes false or misleading information on this form or who omits material or information requested on the form may be subject to criminal sanctions (including fines and imprisonment) and/or civil sanctions (including civil penalties).

PS Form 3526, July 2014 (Page 3 of 4)   PRIVACY NOTICE: See our privacy policy on www.usps.com.

Printed and bound by CPI Group (UK) Ltd, Croydon, CR0 4YY

08/05/2025

01864715-0010